tenminute
workouts

ten minute
workouts

Chrissie Gallagher-Mundy

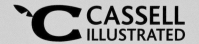
CASSELL
ILLUSTRATED

First published in the United Kingdom in 2003 by Cassell Illustrated,
a division of Octopus Publishing Group Limited
2–4 Heron Quays, London E14 4JP

A CIP catalogue record for this book is available from the British Library

ISBN 1 84403 015 6

Produced and designed by SP Creative Design Ltd
Wickham Skeith, Suffolk, England
Editor: Heather Thomas
Designer: Rolando Ugolini
Jacket design by Jo Knowles
Special photography by Charlie Colmer
Models for photography: personal trainers from The London Academy of
Personal Fitness (www.lapf.co.uk): Sophie Ackroyd, Paul Gunn, Karen
Lamson and Dionne Wright

Printed and bound in Italy

**If you are pregnant or if you have a medical condition
that could be adversely affected by exercise or any doubts
about your health, consult a doctor before embarking on
any exercise programme.**

contents

introduction

Most people, nowadays, realize that they need to keep fit. However, not every one finds it that easy to achieve! Sometimes it can be difficult to know exactly how to go about maintaining fitness on a daily basis. Although there are many different gyms we can join and many different sports we can play to get in shape, we can't always fit in regular sports play and as we get older the problem is often keeping up the consistency. Life, work, socializing, commuting, travel, bringing up children and injuries can all get in the way of regular visits to the gym or sports participation. For those times when you cannot exercise as much as you'd like, it's good to have a home programme that you can do, on your own, without the need of special equipment, and that you can try and keep up week in, week out.

Finding the Right Exercise

There are many toning and stretching exercises that can be done by just using your own body in a small space. Without the need for specialist equipment you can do this kind of programme virtually any time and anywhere. The beauty of this kind of programme is that you can tailor it to suit your needs. You can introduce the kind of exercise you enjoy and you can do it for as long as suits you.

A lot has been written about the intensity and length of time we should exercise. If you are training for a specific event or a competition, then this will dictate the kind of training you need to do. But more often than not, for the average person, training is more about keeping their body ticking over; free from injury and feeling supple and strong. Many people exercise to lose weight and this is a great way to approach weight control, although if you are exercising to burn fat then there is a minimum length of workout you need to be doing. The main thing to remember about a home programme is that it needs to be done consistently. As you work out regularly over a period of time, you will gradually start to feel stronger, fitter, more flexible and supple.

The beauty of this kind of programme is that you can tailor it to suit your needs.

You can introduce the kind of exercise you enjoy and you can do it for as long as suits you.

Finding the Time

One of the keys to doing something consistently is finding the time for it. You have to decide that it is one of your priorities and then make the time in your daily life for it. If exercise becomes something you want to do but never do, it is because you are not really committing mentally and putting aside the time, physically, for it.

There are numerous videos and books as well as organised classes that feature an hour's workout but it doesn't have to last that length of time. Too many people fear that if they don't do an hour's worth of exercise it's not worth doing. This is misguided. Even a small amount of exercise performed regularly over the weeks will make a real difference to your health and well-being.

This is where the programmes in this book will really help you. The exercises are varied and aim to cover all the key elements of fitness, but they are also split into 10-minute blocks. Ten minutes is a block of time that most of us could fit into most of our days. It doesn't sound like long and it needn't be! But done regularly, i.e. every other day (or, ideally, every day), it will make a big difference to your overall feeling of fitness and health.

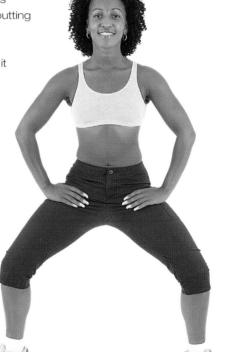

using *this* programme

T his book presents a variety of 10-minute workouts. A 10-minute programme means you should be able to slot a workout like this into even your busiest day! On the following pages, you will read how to deduce which areas you need to focus on and then you can choose your 10-minute blocks accordingly!

Target 10s

There are blocks of 10 aimed at the different areas of your body that you may feel you need to work on and target. You can also use one or two 10s on different days to work together. For example, if you allocate one day to work on your stomachs followed by one day on your hips and thighs and alternate this throughout the week you will be successfully targeting the lower half of your body.

If you want to really improve your shoulders and arms, then alternate these two workouts for a week to target those particular areas. There is also a stretch 10 programme which will keep you supple as you get stronger.

Don't forget that part of an all-round fitness programme includes the areas you can't see – the heart and lungs, i.e. the cardiovascular system. So make sure that at least once in every week you include the CV 10 which will keep you in good stamina shape!

As you get fitter you may find that you want to do more than just 10 minutes at a time. That 10 minutes will soon fly by as you get into the exercise habit! If this is the case, then you can begin to slot two of your 10s together. For instance, you could do the CV 10 followed by a toning 10. This would make for a thorough 20-minute workout.

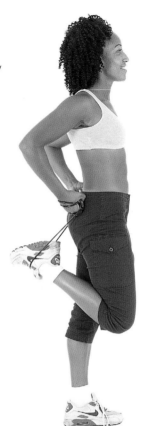

Don't forget that part of an all-round fitness programme includes the areas that you can't see – the heart and lungs, i.e. the cardiovascular system.

Warm Up and Cool Down

At the start of the detailed exercise section of this book, there is a special feature dedicated to warm-up exercises which you should take time to do before you start any of your workouts. The purpose of the warm-up section is to get the body ready for exercise. Warming up is a necessity – every time you exercise. A warm up is exactly what it says; a way of creating heat in the body. As you move, you build heat in the muscles thereby making them more pliable and less prone to tearing or pulling. A warm up should also involve the mobilization of the joints, so that the warmed synovial fluid between the surfaces gives smooth movements and less friction.

The warm-up phase is also a good time to practise with care any of the moves that you might later do at speed. This prepares the body – and the mind – for the action to follow.

Similarly, at the end of the book, there's a cool-down section. The purpose of the cool down is to give your body a chance to wind down from the exercise and to resume its natural rhythm. It also gives your mind the opportunity to refocus and to get ready for the rest of your day. So always try to fit in both the warm up and the cool down sections on either side of your workout 10 every time you exercise.

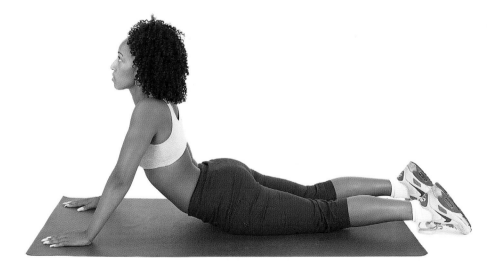

part **1**

understanding

fitness

what is fitness?

We all need to keep fit – it is the modern-day equivalent of having to run and chase an animal to kill and eat it, like our ancestors had to do in order to survive! Actually that is overstating the case a little, but without food we will die, without muscle tone and fitness we will simply run our bodies down and make ourselves more prone to injury and physical problems; and eventually that may damage our health or may even lead to a life-threatening condition!

We are all living longer in this modern age and learning the processes by which we can keep ourselves healthier for longer. One of the most important lessons we must learn is how to keep our bodies fit, supple and free from disease.

Fitness must not be confused with health, however. Someone who is fit may still have health problems and should always take advice from a medical practitioner. Being fit does not mean that you will not get a cold, flu or even that a woman may have an easier time giving birth than someone whom is unfit. What it does mean though is that your recovery time from such events may well be improved.

In the case of some diseases, such as heart disease, high blood pressure and diabetes, regular fitness training can actually help to provide a significant degree of both prevention and treatment for these serious conditions. So put on your gear now and set aside 10 minutes a day to get fit!

fitness components

Fitness or being fit can mean different things to different people. One person may describe it as being able to run for a bus whereas another much older person may describe it as being fit enough to walk round the garden. A man's definition of fitness might be the ability to do 30 push-ups whilst a woman might measure fitness by her capacity to keep dancing for several hours. What all these different descriptions tell us is that fitness is made up of many components. Fitness means having ability in these four key areas:

- Stamina
- Strength and endurance
- Suppleness
- Balance and coordination.

Stamina

This applies to the cardiovascular system. The blood takes energy to the working muscles, enabling our bodies to keep going. This is what we mean by stamina – the ability to keep going. The major players in this scenario are the heart and lungs. The more challenges you give them, the more efficient they become (the heart gets larger and stronger), and the more effort the body can make for a longer period of time. Whilst this was more important when we had to run in order to catch our food – and needed the stamina to chase the buffalo! – we still need stamina today to cope with a busy lifestyle of working, child rearing, stressful commuting and playing sport.

Strength and Endurance

Alongside stamina (or cardiovascular fitness) comes muscular endurance and strength. If muscles don't get used they atrophy, i.e. they wither away. If muscles are used regularly, they will stay toned and shaped. Look at your arms – the chances are that the front of your upper arms are lean and toned. This is because we use our biceps muscles (in the front of the upper arm) constantly to pick up heavy bags and children, etc. If you look at the back of your arms you may see less muscle definition. However, this is because the triceps muscle at the back of the arm only gets used when we do a pushing action – this occurs a lot less frequently in everyday life and therefore the muscle is usually less developed. If, however, you choose to focus on and challenge that particular muscle, then you will notice within weeks that your strength and shape in that area will have increased. The more you work your muscles, the better they work for you.

Nowhere is this more important than in the torso area. If you let your abdominal and back muscles atrophy, your stomach will sag and you may develop problems in the lower back area. Keeping strength and endurance in every muscle leads to a protected and attractive looking body.

Suppleness

Suppleness is about being able to move your body freely. If you are supple, you can perform full ranges of movements in all the joints without pain or strain. Not using your muscles will not only reduce strength but could also affect your ability to perform certain actions. As you exercise, the synovial fluid between the joints is warmed and provides smooth movements. When you stretch regularly, you maintain the flexibility of your muscles so it is important to make stretching a regular part of your routine so that they return to their original length after being tensed. Periods of inaction can lead to muscles becoming shortened and loss of joint mobility. From the age of 30 onwards, muscle tends to reduce in the body and, with it, flexibility. Mature people need to focus on keeping their flexibility as they advance in years.

Balance and Coordination

These are an important part of being fit as they include not just the ability to carry out complicated physical tasks but keeping a correct balance within the body to maintain a good posture. If we lose muscle tone and strength (and gain weight) we may lose coordination. Lack of muscle coordination can lead to injury and can reduce confidence. Staying in touch with your body and listening to it is an important part of maintaining health and fitness. Regular exercise improves our ability to balance and coordinate so we can play sport and keep fit naturally. We can check that the balance of our skeleton is correct by focusing on the postural muscles and keeping them strong.

Combining the Big Four

Ideally, you should combine all these key fitness elements by doing a variety of different activities or exercises. If you focus too much on one activity to the detriment of others, some elements can become overlooked. If you only ever jog, you may miss out on the flexibility element; if you only ever weight-train, you may lack cardiovascular stamina.

Most people are keen to exercise to maintain a general level of fitness for all eventualities, not just for a specific sport. They also want to maintain a good body shape. So when you choose a workout regime and additional sporting activities, make them as varied as possible. This will not only keep your body in peak condition but will give you an attractive, balanced body shape and help to keep you motivated and prevent boredom from setting in.

If you exercise regularly, you will have confidence in your body and it will be less vulnerable to injury. Aim to fit in some form of exercise every other day. If you can't manage this, don't panic – just do as much as you can when you can. The 10-minute workout plan in this book is ideally suited to this philosophy and will still give you good results.

how the programme works

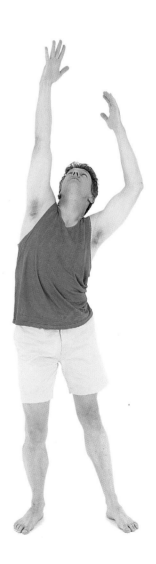

As you begin to do your exercise 10's, you should start to feel a difference. Your muscles will become more toned and stronger and your energy levels should increase. Hopefully, you will begin to get into a rhythm and start to want to do your exercise regularly. The more you do, the more you will want to do. Because each time that you are telling yourself you are only doing 10 minutes you will feel you can always fit it in. As you do this day in, day out, you will reap the benefits.

As your energy level rises, you may also start to feel that you want to do more in other areas of your life. So you can start looking at other ways of adding some more activity into your everyday routine and lifestyle.

Aside from the actual times that you set aside for working out, here are some suggestions on how to include more exercise or action in your everyday life. You may choose not to do all or indeed any of these things, but try to keep them in mind as they will offer you a range of options for increasing your physical activity in simple ways.

Escalate your Activity

Start by assessing exactly how many journeys you make that are less than a mile. How often do you drive these short journeys instead of walking or cycling? Well, why not walk them instead? Walking is more environmentally friendly, it will get you out and about in your local neighbourhood and it will tone you and burn up some extra calories

Why not park a little further away from the shopping centre or mall and do a couple of quick circuits around the mall before you head back to your car?

It may take a little time – planning to factor in an extra 10 minutes of walking time here and there – but that's all it will take, the big 10!

Build up Gradually

Start to factor into your day some little exercise extras. For example, why not try out the following suggestions:

● **Make a stretch start:** try to start your day with a few simple stretches. Why not use the Stretch 10 to get you going in the morning when you step out of bed?

● **Toilet toil:** everyone needs to use the bathroom, several times a day usually, so why not make use of that time and that position? When you squat to lower yourself onto the toilet, repeat that movement away from the toilet! Stand to the side and perform several squats. Finish with a final pulling in on the abdominals to correct your posture.

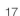

Making an effort to build exercise naturally into your everyday life will bring great fitness rewards and is well worth the effort.

- **Take the most active route possible:** whenever you go out and about, do something physical. A good way to achieve this is to watch some children closely. They are great at getting the most out of every landscape and making it into a playground. If there is something they can climb over, they will! If there is something they can slide under, they will! So take the stairs, not the lift. If there is an escalator, keep walking as it carries you up. If there a railing or fence in your way, step over it – don't walk round it. Sprint for the bus and cycle to work. Do your Stretch 10 as you watch television in the evenings.

how fit are you?

Sometimes it can be difficult to know what is meant by fitness. In the case of Olympic athletes, it is easy to appreciate their fitness as they fly around a racetrack, but what does it mean for the average person? As we said before, fitness is only a part of health, yet it is the part that gives the greatest feeling of *joie de vivre*; the joy of life.

So how do you know if you are fit or unfit? How do you tell if you need to do more? Look at the questions below and answer them as honestly as you can. Just mark a simple 'yes' or 'no' and then check to see how you scored.

Fit or Foe Quiz

1 Do you feel you have enough energy?   YES NO

2 Do you think you could do a 25-metre dash for a bus and still have enough energy left to leap up on the platform at the end?   YES NO

3 Could you lift your own TV set from one side of the room to the other?   YES NO

4 Could you twist right round in a car to see the person behind you?   YES NO

5 Do you exercise more than twice per week?   YES NO

6 Do you walk to several places in an average week?   YES NO

7 Do you have an active hobby, such as a sport or gardening?   YES NO

8 Do you practise some form of relaxation?   YES NO

9 Do you think you need more muscle tone?   YES NO

10 Do you think you need to lose some body fat?   YES NO

11 Do you think your body looks flabby?   YES NO

12 Are you unhappy with your body shape?   YES NO

Interpreting your answers

Questions 1–4

The first four questions in our lifestyle quiz relate to the confidence you gain if you are fit. If you are feeling fit then you will have confidence in your body's ability to do what it needs for you at any given moment. You will feel ready (physically) for most things and if, for instance, you suddenly had to run for a bus, you would not be worrying about whether your heart and legs would get you there!

If you answered mostly 'no' to these four questions, then you may feel that you need to do some work in order to get fitter.

Questions 5–8

These four questions relate to the level of activity you are already doing. The more we do, the more we feel like doing. The body responds to regular activity and exercise by becoming stronger and more flexible to cope with these demands.

If you answered mostly 'no' to these four questions you definitely need to increase your activity level and put in some regular exercise sessions to keep your body in top form.

Questions 9–12

These four questions relate to how your body looks. We often judge how fit people are by the way they look. Although this isn't always the case, people who are active and strong usually show it in the shape and muscle tone of their bodies.

If you answered mostly 'yes' to these last four questions, then you are probably a little unhappy with your figure. We all have times when we feel that we could look better, but if this is merely just a case of doing some exercises for body toning and shaping then don't sit around and fret – get going! With just 10 minutes a day, you can start to make a difference to your body and gain confidence in your physical abilities and shape.

working towards fitness

So what are realistic aims when you are trying to get fit? The key thing to remember when trying to increase your level of fitness is to take it slowly. The most frustrating thing about changing the body, whether it is losing weight or gaining strength, is that it doesn't happen overnight. It is a gradual process and you have to work at it and be patient.

It is the same when learning a new sport or even a new discipline, such as using a new computer programme; you have to do a little each day and add more to the routine as the weeks go by. Eventually, you will reap the benefits of this sensible approach.

It really is the old adage that makes sense here: practice makes perfect. Building muscle tone doesn't happen overnight – it can take six weeks or more – and losing body fat can take at least a similar amount of time before any significant loss can be seen.

For many people, this slow process is just too much and this has resulted in a fitness and health industry that is forever offering people quick fixes. There are potions and pills galore for weight loss. There are gadgets and gimmicks that promise a body shape change almost instantly.

Similarly, even some gyms promise amazing results in unrealistic time frames and this can lead to the 'all or nothing' mentality. Many people join a gym enthusiastically with the best intentions and work out four or even five times a week in the first three weeks. However, this makes them sore, tired and can even cause injuries and, after the initial love affair, they often become unfocused, unenthusiastic and stop going.

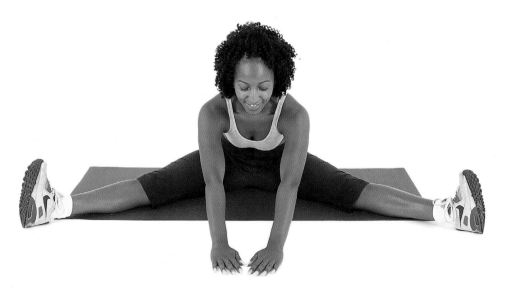

The best kind of fitness programme,
if you can do it, is as follows:

- The kind that starts slowly and builds.
- A programme that you can follow at home is all the better because there is more chance of you doing it regularly.
- A programme that starts with some very basic moves and then adds a few new ones each day.
- A fitness regime that leaves you feeling challenged by your routine but you are not shattered at the end of it.
- A routine that you should look forward to fitting into your day as a chance to relax mentally and stretch yourself physically.
- A programme that may leave you feeling slightly stiff in the first few days, but after that simply revitalized and ready to go!

types of fitness

There are several types of fitness, as we have already discovered. In the following pages, you will find more detailed information on what each one means and how best you can achieve it.

Cardiovascular Fitness

When we speak of cardiovascualr fitness we generally refer to the type of exercise that uses the heart and lungs and therefore means we are breathing more heavily than normal. Most exercise is either aerobic or anaerobic (*see* opposite). Both terms refer to the energy system that the body uses when doing different types of exercise. Both types of exercise use energy sources in different ways and make different demands on the body.

What is Aerobic Exercise?

Aerobic exercises essentially mean 'with air' so that the body uses oxygen to metabolize stored fat into energy. Aerobic exercise is characterized by the fact that you would be using large muscle groups, rhythmically, for a period of 20 minutes or longer and that you would be breathing fairly heavily. At this point the body needs to metabolize the stored energy into the bloodstream in order to keep the activity going. So fat is taken from storage and converted to energy to be transported around the body.

So what is aerobic exercise? In a nutshell, it is the different types of rhythmic exercise that use large muscle groups with the body, such as running, cycling, rowing, walking and skating. It has the following characteristics:

- Relatively medium exertion intensity: if you are working too hard, you won't be able to keep going for 20 minutes.
- Rhythmic work so that the body relaxes into it: a good example of this type of aerobic activity is cross-country skiing where the muscles or limbs aren't over-stressed.
- Variety of movement: if this isn't possible as, for example, with running, then vary your views and environment so that you're not too bored to keep going for 20 minutes plus.
- Your breathing should be regular and not gasping but your heart will be pumping relatively hard.

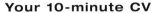

Your 10-minute CV

Try to perform your CV (cardiovascular) section regularly, i.e. two to three times a week. This will ensure that you are starting to push your heart a little. The reason why many people have poor cardiovascular fitness (the ability to keep going) is that most activities they do in their daily life do not push their heart in any sustained way, and therefore the heart remains unchallenged. If you challenge it, then like any other muscle, it will increase in size and performance to meet the challenge.

Make sure as you do the CV 10 that you are breathing quite heavily. The workout should feel harder work than a casual walk or swim, but you should still be able to carry on a conversation as you exercise. If you are alone, sing to yourself! This will ensure that you are not working too hard. If you push your heart too hard, then your exercise will not remain aerobic but become anaerobic (*see* opposite).

If you are exercising to reduce stored body fat you will need to go beyond the 10-minute programme presented on pages 98–105. You need to work towards a 20- or 30-minute period, and then you know your body will be delving into your fat stores just to keep moving. Add two or three of your CV 10s together to achieve this.

23

If you challenge your heart, then like any other muscle, it will increase in size and performance to meet the challenge.

toning fitness

Whereas cardiovascular exercise works and tones the heart and lungs, toning exercise contracts the muscles against resistance. When you lift a bag off the ground or, indeed, perform any kind of movement, the muscles contract and pull on the bones. As you tone the muscles, you stress them, and it this stress that stimulates them to increase in size and shape in order to cope with the extra demands.

As we move around we are continuously contracting and relaxing our muscles. However, if you want to tone a specific muscle group then it is best to contract the muscle against resistance. This might mean lifting something heavy so that the muscle has to work hard by pushing against, or pulling on, something. When you do regular, rhythmic toning exercise, you are using a different energy system from the one you employ when performing your cardiovascular training. When you tone and work your muscles, you are using the glycogen already available in them. When this energy in the muscles begins to run low, you start to feel a burning, aching sensation, which is a by-product called lactic acid, in your muscles. This will cause the affected muscle to ache and will make you stop the exercise temporarily.

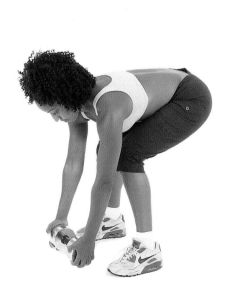

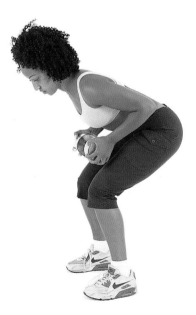

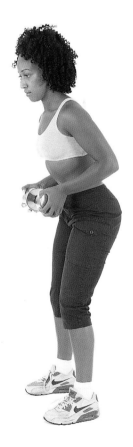

What is Toning Exercise?

Toning exercise is any movement that contracts the muscles against force. This includes lifting heavy things, lifting your own body weight, or pushing or pulling on something heavy. There are different levels and intensities of toning exercise with various characteristics.

- It can be maximum-exertion intensity. When the muscles get tired and the energy starts to run out, you will feel the 'burn'!
- It can be sporadic activity where the body works hard one minute and stops the next. Examples of this would include tennis, squash, football and other similar sports.
- It can be a whole variety of movement routines, which include weight lifting, Dynaband pulling, lifting your own body weight and even activities such as gardening which can be toning on the muscles!
- Your breathing will be fairly regular but there may be times, for instance when lifting weights, when you will breathe more forcefully.

25

Your 10-minute Toners

Try to perform the exercises in the toning section regularly, i.e. twice a week. Muscles need to be worked; otherwise they atrophy and disappear – so keep up the pumping! When you do a toning routine you will feel the ache of lactic acid (where the energy has run low), so take a brief rest and then continue.

After you have completed a tough toning routine you may well feel stiff for a day or so after the exercise. If this is the case, then take a hot shower, warm up and do a couple of stretches or, if the stiffness is really bad, take an aspirin (if it is medically safe for you to do so – if in doubt, check with your doctor). As you exercise more regularly and become fitter and more supple, the stiffness will decline.

When you perform a toning routine you can decide which areas you specifically want to tone. The more that you work a muscle, the stronger and larger and more shapely it will become. Choose from the variety of toning 10s in this book and focus on whichever area of your body needs most work!

As you exercise more regularly and become fitter and more supple, the stiffness will decline.

stretching fitness

The stretching part of your overall fitness routine is all about lengthening the muscles. The only problem with doing all the toning and cardiovascular exercises is that as well as strengthening the muscles (of the heart and body) you can also make them tight. As you contract and release the muscles against resistance, the force of the contraction causes microscopic tears, which are believed to cause stiffness. These are subsequently repaired by the body to create stronger, more fibrous muscle. As the muscle rebuilds, it will tighten, and if you do not take the time and care to stretch it back to its original length you may find that your flexibility of movement decreases.

There is also a second phase of stretching in which you can work towards increasing your flexibility. This may involve holding the stretch positions for longer to get the muscle to release further. This kind of stretching can improve alignment and help extend your range of flexibility and mobility. It is also thought to aid the muscle's recovery from the toning phase and lessen the effects of stiffness.

Things to Remember When Stretching

Basically, all stretching exercise involves the following:
- A movement that extends the muscle and allows it to return to its pre-exercised, original length state.
- There are many different ways of effecting a stretch. The most important factor to remember, however, is that you must be warm before you can stretch. So always do your stretching at the end of a session of exercise, not at the beginning when your body will be too cold to be able to stretch safely.
- Some stretches may be included as part of your warm-up session. However, these should generally be active stretches, such as where you kick your foot out to extend the leg. This will actively stretch the hamstring. These types of stretches simply act as a rehearsal for some of the moves you may do in the main body of your routine.
- Stretches can be held just for a short period to simply return the muscle to its pre-exercise length or, alternatively, they may be held for longer. This can be done alone or with a partner to aid you in developing the stretch. This is known as developmental stretching.
- Stretching can also be performed using a technique called PNF where you use the contraction of the opposing muscles to stretch the target muscle even further.

There really is a whole variety of ways by which you can work on increasing your flexibility and range of movement. If this is your particular interest, after practising the stretches outlined in this book, you may wish to follow a full stretch plan which you can take further. For example, many dance routines work on stretching, as does yoga.

It is important that you breathe evenly and rhythmically throughout any kind of stretching routine. Never hold your breath or strain but try to use the outward breath to take the stretch a little further.

Your 10-minute Stretch

Stretching should be done weekly at the very least. Ideally, you should try to do some shorter stretches at the end of each 10-minute routine to lengthen the muscles that you use and to minimize any stiffness

If your goal, on a certain day, is to increase your flexibility, then choose a very active 10 so that you are really warm before you begin to stretch. The more warmth in the body the better the synovial fluid works over the joints, and the more inclined the muscles are to lengthen.

When you are stretching, you should feel your muscles pulling slightly. Hold this position, whilst continuing to breathe normally, and then take it a little further if it feels comfortable to do so.

Whilst stretching out tight areas you may feel some mild discomfort but you should not feel great pain. If this happens, then stop immediately. Do not try to force your body; instead, hold a position until you feel the muscle start to give up and then relax.

Always try to do your stretching when you are warm or sweating. Stretch in a warm room, and keep some extra clothes handy to pile on the layers if you start to feel cool.

27

The more warmth in the body the better the synovial fluid works over the joints, and the more inclined the muscles are to lengthen.

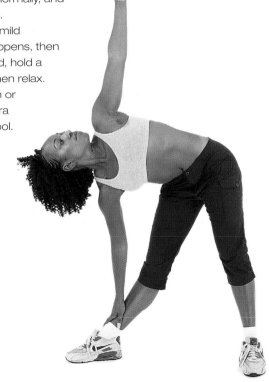

make the programme work your way

The following programme of routine 10s is very flexible. You can choose any areas you like to focus on. You can also combine the 10s in different combinations and at different times during the week to make sure that you cover every aspect of fitness.

Remember that the main aim for all-round fitness is variety! Variety of movement and variety of discipline will keep you interested and keep your body guessing, too. The less repetitive your successive workouts are, the less prone you will be to injury and boredom.

To begin with you, will need to start slowly and work up gradually. Even 10 minutes will make you stiff and sore if you approach it wrongly. So after doing your first 10 minutes on Day 1, you should rest on Day 2. It is important to build a programme slowly and the best way to do this is by starting with a little and then adding to what you did the first day the following time you exercise. If you build up slowly but regularly, your workouts will become more challenging without you having to think about it!

Workout Plans

Use the examples below to build your own combinations. They are included as illustrations to give you an idea of how to increase the level at which you work.

1 Beginner's level

Day 1	Warm up	Hips and thighs
Day 2	Rest	
Day 3	Warm up	Hips and thighs
Day 4	Rest	
Day 5	Warm up	Shoulders and arms

In this example for beginners, you are giving your body a chance to get used to the moves in the first week before you add something new. It also enables you to cover the large muscles of the body and give them a good workout.

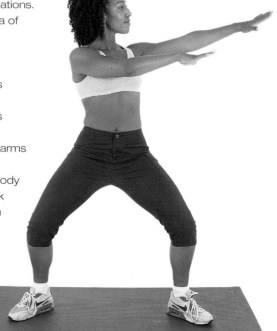

2 Moving on

Day 1	Warm up	Hips and thighs
Day 2	Rest	
Day 3	Warm up	Shoulders and arms
Day 4	Rest	
Day 5	Warm up	Abdominals
Day 6	Rest	
Day 7	Warm up	Stretch top to toe

Here you are starting to build on what you have achieved in the beginner's workout by increasing the pace at which you exercise and by working out other areas of the body.

3 Really keen

Day 1	Warm up	Hips and thighs/Arms
Day 2	warm up	Stretch
Day 3	Warm up	Abdominals/Back and shoulders
Day 4	Rest	
Day 5	Warm up	CV/ Stretch top to toe

By the time you reach this level, you will have really increased the workload and you are also covering all the major muscles and all your fitness needs in this week's workout.

4 Spot specific

Day 1	Warm up	Hips and thighs
Day 2	Warm up	Abdominals
Day 3	Warm up	Hips and thighs
Day 4	Warm up	Abdominals
Day 5	Warm up	Hips and thighs/Stretch

Here you have built a programme that targets your lower body. In the second week, you might well add in the CV 10 to the mix to increase the intensity further. When you have shaped up your lower half, you can swap the 10s around to even up the workload again. Remember: any way you want to fit the pieces together, this workout can be personalized to work for you!

eat towards fitness

Although there is much conflicting advice around on what to eat and how to eat it, there is a current consensus on the kinds of food that make a positive difference to your health and diet. The guidelines below will stand you in good stead for a healthy eating plan to go with your healthy workout routines. If you don't always stick to these suggestions, don't panic, but do try to keep to these principles 80 per cent of the time.

Eat Little and Often

It is important when you are trying to tone up, burn body fat and lead a healthy existence that you eat regularly. If you go for long periods without eating you will not have the energy you need to sustain you throughout the ups and downs of your daily routine. If you are now doing regular exercise, you need to make sure that your body has the fuel it needs to keep going. Regular eating will keep your blood sugar levels up and your mood elevated.

People who restrict their food intake too much can find that their body acts as though there may be starvation on the horizon and starts to conserve body fat. It also starts to conserve energy and slows down the metabolism. So they find it increasingly hard to lose weight and also feel low in energy.

After an exercise session in which you have worked your muscles and used up the glycogen (sugars), your body needs food to replenish its stores and to enable it to rebuild muscle tissue. If you do not eat for long periods after exercising you may be reducing your ability to build muscle tone – the very thing that you are trying to achieve.

Eating little and often, instead of one large meal a day, will aid your digestion, raise your energy levels and help muscle tone. So you don't need to eat big meals and really pile your plate up; try grazing through the day with smaller meals and some really healthy, nutritious snacks of fruit and raw vegetables. Don't forget that your metabolism is raised after exercise so now is the time to eat healthily and heartily! Read the following pages for some helpful advice on how to do it.

If you are now doing regular exercise, you need to make sure that your body has the fuel it needs to keep going.

Eat a Low-fat Diet

When you over-eat, it doesn't matter whether you have eaten fat, carbohydrate or protein – the excess will still be stored, under the skin, as fat. Whilst some fat in the diet is beneficial, there are, however, two very good reasons to eat a diet which is relatively low in fat.

The fat that we eat has far more calories per gram (9 calories) than protein (4 calories) or carbohydrates (4 calories). So if you are trying to restrict your calories, remember that you can eat more carbohydrates and protein and clock up less calories in a day than if your diet relies too heavily on fats. In other words, you can eat many more plates of vegetables or fruit before clocking up 300 calories than packets of crisps. So if eating is your pleasure, eat things that you can eat a lot of!

A diet that is too high in fat (particularly saturated fat) is known to contribute to coating, thereby restricting the width of the arteries and veins, and this, of course, can be a contributory factor in causing heart problems.

31

Eat vegetables and fruit

The golden rule for healthy eating is every time you have a plate of food, try to make sure that there are some fruit or vegetables on it! This is relatively easy to achieve in your everyday life if you follow these simple guidelines. Current nutritional advice states that we should all try to eat at least five portions of fresh vegetables or fruit every day. Here's how.

Breakfast When you eat breakfast – and this is probably the most important meal of the day so don't be tempted to skip it – try to ensure there are some strawberries or other fruit mixed in with your cereal or some slices of peach or kiwi alongside your porridge or some fresh cherries or blueberries baked in with your muffins.

Lunch When eating lunch, make sure that the majority of your plate is covered in salad or vegetables or beans or pulses. Don't snack on crisps, chocolate or fatty foods, such as pastries and cookies. And, instead of a dessert, treat yourself to a piece of fruit or a fresh fruit salad.

Dinner When you eat your evening meal, mix some beans in with your accompanying rice or some sweet corn amongst your pasta or some spring onions and cabbage into your mashed potato. Always try to eat some green vegetables or a salad with your main course. If you eat potatoes, have them baked in their skins or boiled rather than fried or roasted in fat.

Benefits of Vegetables and Fruit

Vegetables and fruit contain important vitamins, minerals and other nutrients that our bodies require, so they should be a nutritional priority. Try to ensure these make up the majority of your diet – this is easily done by making them the largest portion on your plate! A diet that is rich in fruit and vegetables is thought to help guard against carcinogens, which cause cancer, arthritis and many other illnesses, including heart disease.

They are also great foods when it comes to fat loss. They supply excellent energy in the form of complex carbohydrates and are low in both calories and fat. This means you can eat far more of them and so feel comfortably full and satisfied without putting in excess calories. In addition to all this, fruit can be enjoyed at any time of the day, whether you're at work or relaxing at home.

- Bananas are a particularly portable and edible fruit and are a really fast energy source, so when you exercise keep one handy!
- Carry canned tinned fruits (in natural juice, not syrup) with you as handy, juicy pick-me-ups.
- Frozen vegetables and fruit are equally good for you – and the frozen packet can help with the odd injury, too, when you need to apply some ice!

Whole Grains

Whole wheat and rice products provide the complex carbohydrates that our bodies need to keep the blood concentration balanced. So try to include whole-grain breads, breakfast cereals, pasta and rice on your plate once a day. You don't need to go to a health food store or specialist shop to buy these; all supermarket chains sell them.

Avoid Sugar and Salt

Too much sugar leads to too much fluctuation in the blood sugar levels in the body as well as storage of fat. This, in turn, can eventually lead to an onset of diabetes and other health problems later in life. Sugar is a hidden, invisible ingredient in many of the foods we eat and you may not even realize that it is lurking in biscuits, cookies, cakes, confectionery, baked beans, many sauces and ready meals, and popular soft drinks and mixers. Read the labels carefully to check the sugar content before you buy them.

You can reduce sugar in your diet by substituting some honey or dried or natural fruits when cooking; by changing to an artificial sweetener; opting for low-calorie soft drinks; and cutting down on processed foods and snacks which tend to have a high sugar content.

Too much salt has been linked to stomach cancer and is thought to raise blood pressure so try to restrict your salt intake. We all need some salt for good health but sodium is present in most of the foods we eat and it should not be necessary to add salt to food at the table after cooking. To cut down on salt, add only a small amount when cooking (usually half the amount that the recipe states); substitute herbs and spices as alternative seasonings; or use a low-sodium substitute that will still provide the taste.

Water

Try to drink at least eight to ten glasses of water per day. Dehydration can occur without us becoming aware of it. If you are thirsty you are already dehydrated and although you may feel better after several sips your body needs much, much more. Dehydration can adversely affect your posture, your energy levels and your hunger levels. It also lowers the metabolism by two to three per cent.

Many people claim that water is boring and tasteless and that they prefer soft drinks or juice. If you feel like this, then try some different types of bottled water and add fresh fruit juice for a quick refresher after a workout! If you always keep a bottle of water handy throughout the day and sip rather than glug back a whole pint at once, then you won't be rushing to the toilet every five minutes!

Bottled water can be quite expensive if you drink a lot of it. The latest research shows that tap water is probably just as good for you so don't worry if you can't afford the bottled sort. Alternatively, you may wish to invest in a water filter and keep some water handy in the refrigerator at all times.

Alcohol

Whilst some studies suggest that a glass of red wine may be beneficial to our blood pressure, there is not much goodness in alcohol, particularly if you are watching your weight. We know that it is a great relaxant and socializer and it is impractical to suggest that you should never touch another drop, but remember the maxim: as little as humanly possible! Alcohol, of any description, does three devastating things for the health-conscious person:

- It turns off your appetite switch: When you drink, you cease to notice what you are putting in to your body. As the alcohol influences you, it can turn off your natural 'I've had enough' switch so that you don't notice you are full and you keep on eating. Not only does this leave you feeling stuffed and ill but you have significantly overloaded your calories.
- It turns on your fat storing cells: Alcohol is not used in the body for any healthy process. If you take in fat, carbohydrates or proteins they are used for important functions, yet alcohol is regarded as a toxin by the body and it spends its time trying to expel it. Also, the sugar that comes from alcohol, if it is not used up immediately, is stored as fat. Not only this but it primes your cells to store more fat!
- It turns off your will power to exercise and be sensible about eating.

If you have spent days working on toning your muscles and slenderizing your shape, don't ruin your next day's progress with one alcohol blitz. Keep a track on your intake and don't drink till you feel fuzzy because after a few glasses you will start to say: ' Hey, I don't care if I don't stick to my eating/exercising plan any more' or 'What does it matter if I have one blow out tonight? Can't a guy enjoy himself?' However, remember that the next morning you will care and you'll wish you hadn't done it! So avoid the drink and don't do it!

the mental approach

When keeping up an exercise routine, one of the most important things is keeping your momentum going. Too many times people join gyms, take up classes and go full pelt on the running track, only to lose their enthusiasm three weeks later. The all or nothing syndrome provides the fitness industry's constant supply of clients but, sadly, it also fills the injury waiting rooms of physiotherapists, doctors and diet quacks.

When you approach your programme try to be realistic about how and when you can do it. Do not perform all the 10-minute routines listed in this book joined together in your first week! All you will do is make yourself stiff and sore and it will put you off doing anything during the next few days. Start slowly and build up gradually as suggested on page 28.

Manage Your Time

If you decide that keeping fit is going to be a regular part of your life, then you need to make time for it. Set aside a regular slot for your 10-minute routine. The most regular exercisers find that working out in the morning is best. In this way, you can do your workout early on in the day when you have lots of energy and then it's over and you don't need to worry. There may be days, however, when early morning won't work. Later in the day you may also feel more awake and less stiff. It's probably best to keep the arrangement as flexible as possible. Perhaps aim to do your workout most mornings but don't be rigid about it. For instance, if you don't have time earlier in the day, you can always fit it in before you go to bed if that's the only time you have.

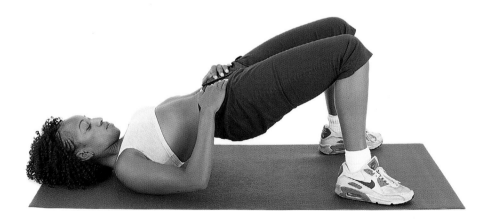

If you decide that keeping fit is going to be a regular part of your life, then you need to make time for it.

If you miss a day here and there – or even several days – don't get disheartened and give up. There may be times when you are too busy but you shouldn't feel as though there is no point in carrying on because there is! Even if you miss a week of exercise every so often, if the majority of the time you have kept at it, it will still make a difference and you will retain an element of fitness. A little exercise even on an irregular basis is better than none at all.

We all have times when we feel de-motivated or when there are other things in our life to distract us and take precedence. It's hard to have getting fit at the top of your priority list the whole time, and it's also impractical. To make this programme work effectively, it has to become a natural and automatic part of your daily or every-other-daily ritual – not a special programme which you make a special effort to do. Then it will be like brushing your teeth or combing your hair each day; 10 minutes that you don't even have to think about!

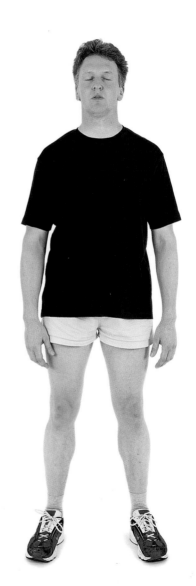

relaxation
and stress

One of the major benefits of a regular exercise routine is not only the effect that it has on the body but also on the mind. Modern life carries so many stresses and strains that the mind can become overburdened. As we worry, fret and simply run over problems in our minds, our thoughts tend to run over the same patterns and the same thoughts. Giving the mind a chance to focus on something completely different which absorbs the mind can then leave it feeling refreshed at the end of a session. We all have our own ways of dealing with stress and these vary between individuals. Some people, for instance, find that walking, gardening or some other leisure pursuit or hobby relaxes them and absorbs their attention. These are all good ideas yet exercise has the potential to be even more stress-releasing because you are working with your own body.

Putting aside some time to exercise and really concentrating on what you are doing will increase the rewards of your workout for both your body and your mind. Before you are aware of it, 10 minutes will have flown by and you won't have thought of anything else but your exercises! When you have a busy, stressful day, this is almost like taking a 10-minute nap for your mind!

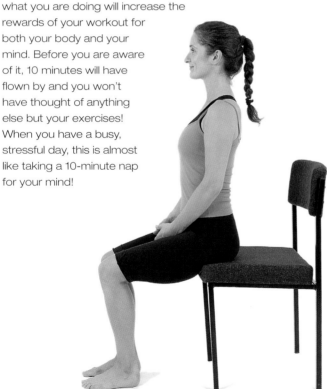
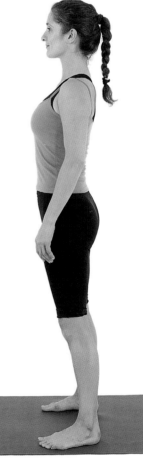

10-minute Mind Nap

In order to achieve a real mind nap, select a simple workout routine with which you are familiar and can relax into automatically without much thought.

Instructions

1 Make sure you can run through the exercises without having to think too much about what comes next.

2 Now start to work through your chosen routine and really think about each step that you take.

3 Perform each movement more slowly and carefully than normal.

4 Try to concentrate solely on what you are doing, and where each body part should go in relation to the other and how each move feels.

5 When you are in any given position, think about what muscle you are using to effect the move. The more you focus on the muscle the more effectively you will perform the exercise.

6 Keep a constant check on your posture even when you are not exercising. For correct posture, see the photographs on the opposite page.

- Check that your abdominals are pulled in and lifted to support the back.
- Check that your shoulders are down, not hunched up around your ears.
- Check that your tail bone is pulling down towards the floor.
- When you are standing, the top of your head should be pressing towards the ceiling.
- When you are sitting, you should keep your ribcage lifted and your back as erect as possible.

7 Think about your breathing; try to keep it regular – don't hold your breath but breathe deeply and rhythmically when making an effort.

8 Try to register what your body is feeling in each position:

- Does it feel comfortable?
- At what point does the burn (lactic acid) kick in?
- Are you doing the move with a full range of movement?

9 The more you concentrate on exactly what you are doing, the more your mind will release its usual paths of thought. Therefore when you finish your routine not only will you have done a particularly effective workout but your mind will be refreshed, too!

37

alexander 10:
de-stress your body

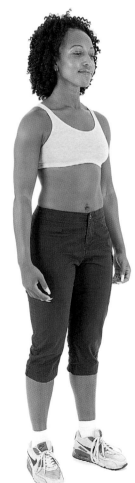

As we have seen, regular exercise can help both the mind and the body, but this is not the only way in which we can help ourselves towards a more relaxed lifestyle. How we carry out our daily tasks is an area that we can improve and bring a new approach to both mentally and physically.

In all areas of our lives we can become aware of where minor stresses and strains occur. Sometimes we need to understand that less is more, and that tasks can be more effectively and calmly accomplished by simple movement and thought. The mind and body are intimately connected, and thus problems in our everyday lives can be transformed into habit-forming physical tensions. However, if we can learn to release the physical side of us, we can also help the mental part of us to cope better. In this way, we can think more calmly and move in a more efficient and beneficial way.

Using the Alexander technique, students are encouraged to make full use of the body's natural alignment and balance. This balance is all too often ignored or over-ruled in pursuit of our busy, modern-day lifestyle when we are always short of time and rushing around trying to fit everything in. Slowing down enough to recap on the body's natural resources can be very important.

We are always short of time and rushing around trying to fit everything in. Slowing down enough to recap on the body's natural resources can be very important.

Relaxing Alexander Phrases

Try the following Alexander phrases to relax your movement and your posture. Start by putting aside 10 minutes to focus on some of the Alexander technique commands. These focus the mind on an area of tension without actually doing anything to it.

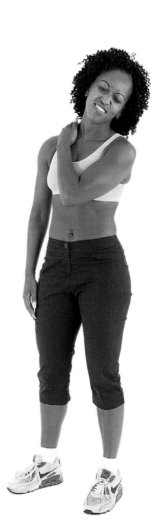

1 Start by standing and thinking your way through your body. Don't tell your body to do anything different. Just note where there is tension, and where there seems to be any imbalance of weight but don't readjust. Alexander stresses the value of first inhibiting habits rather than just overlaying them with new ones. When you have noticed tensions in your body you can start to think about inhibiting the habitual reactions that normally occur.

2 Now, without making any changes, just think through some of the following phrases:
- Neck release: 'Head forwards and up'. Don't thrust your neck forwards or back in an effort to carry out this thought; simply let it rest in the mind making minute physiological changes.
- Now think: 'Back lengthen and widen'. In this way you are not pushing your body into severe postures, as in 'Back straight, stomach in'. Yet you are suggesting to your body a concept – that of your muscles lengthening and widening at the same time. Therefore there is no greater pull on one area or another of your body.
- Now think: 'Shoulders releasing and widening'.
- If you bend your knees think: 'Knees forward and away over the toes'.

Remember that the main stable working areas of the body are the trunk and pelvis, both of which are strong and flexible. Above this is the head.

3 You should sit freely and without any tension as these thoughts help your body to relax. As you work through the phrases above you may feel your body relaxing and rejuvenating a little.

And now that you are relaxed, it is time to start the real 10s!

before you get started

M ake sure before you start any workout programme that you are fit enough to exercise. This means not only preparing for it physically but mentally as well. It is sensible to consider the following points before you begin to ensure that you gain the maximum benefit from the workout.

The Workout Space
First of all, check out the space in which you will be working. Ideally, you need a room with enough space to take at least *five* large steps in either direction.
- Check for any obstacles that may be in the way and remove them.
- Check that there is a window which you can open for ventilation as you begin to sweat!
- Check that the room has a carpet or, better still, an exercise mat for your floor work.
- Check that you have a stereo system or CD player on which you can play some different types of music to influence and improve your routine.

Warm Up First
It is very important, even if your workout is just 10 minutes, that you warm up thoroughly before each session. You can use the warm-up routines in this book (*see* page 44) or even devise some special ones of your own. Gentle jogging or brisk walking around your neighbour hood or a nearby park or even a really fast swim would also warm you up.

What to Wear
To help build up warmth in your body, you should also begin your routine wearing some layers of clothes. Wear something loose and soft in a breathable fabric (there are many choices nowadays). You might choose, for example, a vest with a sweatshirt over the top and some shorts covered with sweat pants. As you get warmer while you work out, you can begin stripping off the layers to keep a comfortable temperature. Starting with more clothes on will retain your body heat when you need it at the beginning and help guard against injury.

Check with Your Doctor

If you have not exercised for some time or suffer from any kind of health problem or complication, it would be sensible to check with your doctor that he or she feels that it is appropriate for you to pursue an unsupervised exercise programme. If you are overweight, your doctor may well encourage you to start exercising as soon as possible, but you should get your blood pressure checked and start exercising gradually and gently.

Working with Weights

There are several exercises in the workout 10s that require the use of weights. Your best buy is probably a pair of dumbbells. They do, however, need to be the right weight to be effective. In order to calculate this, you need to work out your 10 rep maximum.

How to find your 10 rep max.

In order to do this you need to work with a variety of weights so go to your local gym or sports store and perform a bicep curl.

1 Stand straight, holding a weight in one hand, which is turned in towards your thigh.

2 Contract the bicep muscle at the front of your arm and turn the palm in towards the arm as you bend the arm.

3 Slowly lower the arm back down again.

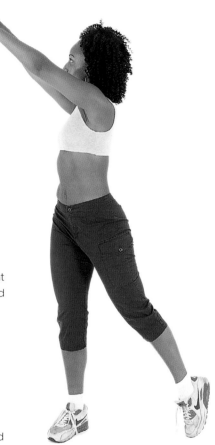

41

Repeat this basic bicep curl experiment with a range of different weights until you find a weight that you can do 10 repetitions with – but only 10! At repetition 9 or 10 your muscles should feel tired, as if you can't do any more. If you can do 15 or 20 repetitions easily with a weight, then it's too light and you must experiment with some others to find the right one for you. When you can do 10 repetitions, and only just 10, you have found your 10-rep max. This will ensure that you are working with a weight which is heavy enough to really tone your body.

part 2

the
ten

minute workouts

warm up

To perform some simple toning exercises it is not necessary to go through a really long warm-up routine. However, creating some warmth in your body and just mobilizing your joints a little will allow you to perform the different workout exercises more effectively and safely. Put some music on and use these movements to move around and create some heat and energy in your body.

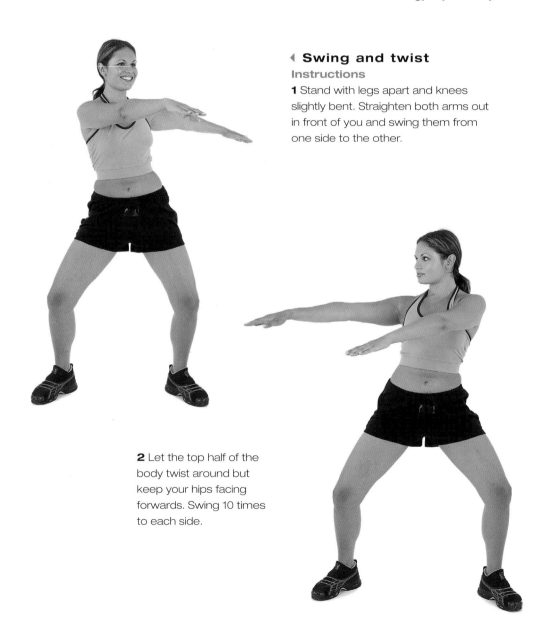

◀ **Swing and twist**

Instructions

1 Stand with legs apart and knees slightly bent. Straighten both arms out in front of you and swing them from one side to the other.

2 Let the top half of the body twist around but keep your hips facing forwards. Swing 10 times to each side.

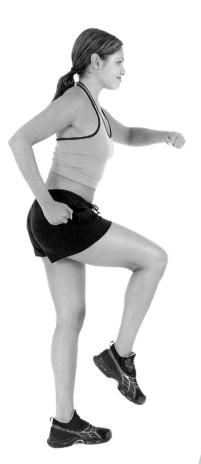

◀ Marching
Instructions
March on the spot, swinging your arms and lifting your knees up as high as you can for 2–3 minutes.

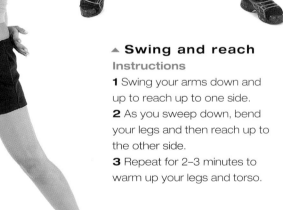

▶ Twisting
Instructions
Swing your arms around your body from side to side, so that your torso twists and your arms wrap around your body. This will warm up your torso and waist. Repeat for 2–3 minutes.

▲ Swing and reach
Instructions
1 Swing your arms down and up to reach up to one side.
2 As you sweep down, bend your legs and then reach up to the other side.
3 Repeat for 2–3 minutes to warm up your legs and torso.

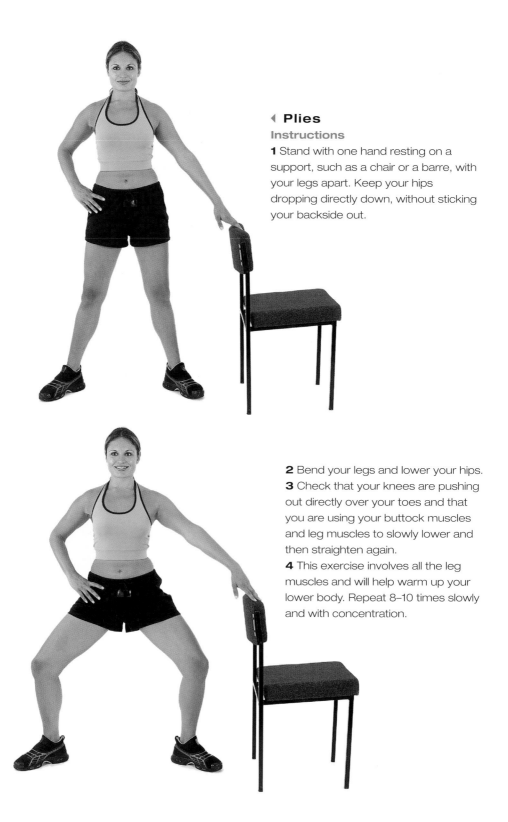

◀ Plies

Instructions

1 Stand with one hand resting on a support, such as a chair or a barre, with your legs apart. Keep your hips dropping directly down, without sticking your backside out.

2 Bend your legs and lower your hips.
3 Check that your knees are pushing out directly over your toes and that you are using your buttock muscles and leg muscles to slowly lower and then straighten again.
4 This exercise involves all the leg muscles and will help warm up your lower body. Repeat 8–10 times slowly and with concentration.

▶ Leg swings

Instructions

1 Stand with one hand resting on a support, such as a chair or barre, and balance on one leg with the knee bent.
2 Now pull yourself up in your supporting hip so that you stand tall and aligned.

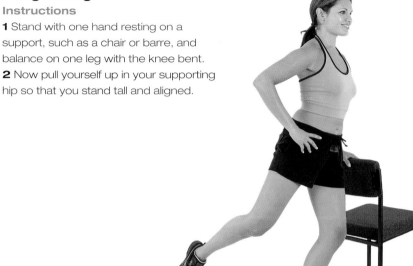

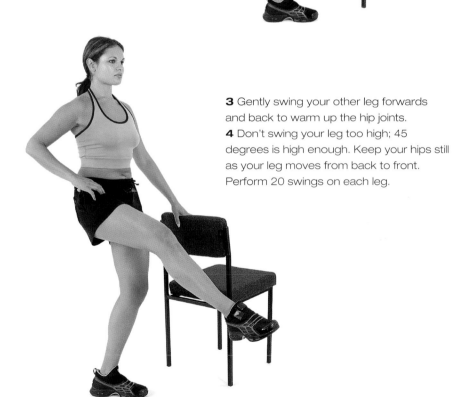

3 Gently swing your other leg forwards and back to warm up the hip joints.
4 Don't swing your leg too high; 45 degrees is high enough. Keep your hips still as your leg moves from back to front. Perform 20 swings on each leg.

arm workout

Some parts of your arms will stay naturally toned as a result of carrying out everyday tasks and actions. The forearms tend not to amass body fat and stay lean and muscular. It is the bicep muscle at the front of the arm and the tricep muscle at the back that need toning in order to shape and improve the sight of your arms in a short-sleeved or sleeveless top! Use these exercises to tone and firm the upper arms.

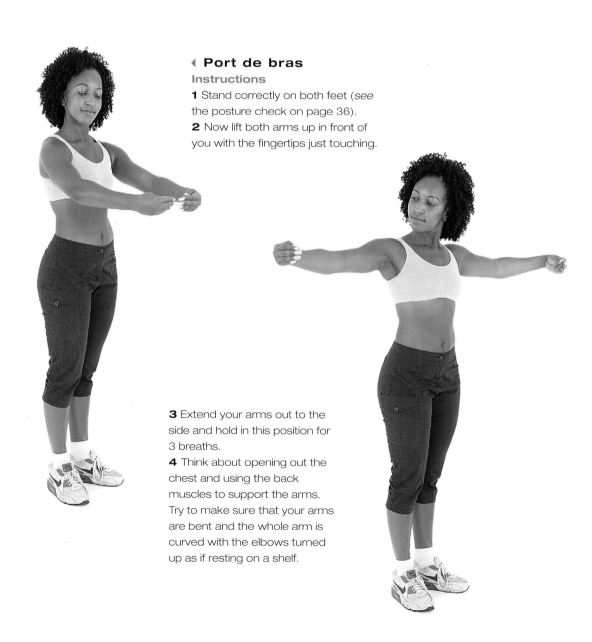

◀ **Port de bras**

Instructions

1 Stand correctly on both feet (*see* the posture check on page 36).
2 Now lift both arms up in front of you with the fingertips just touching.

3 Extend your arms out to the side and hold in this position for 3 breaths.
4 Think about opening out the chest and using the back muscles to support the arms. Try to make sure that your arms are bent and the whole arm is curved with the elbows turned up as if resting on a shelf.

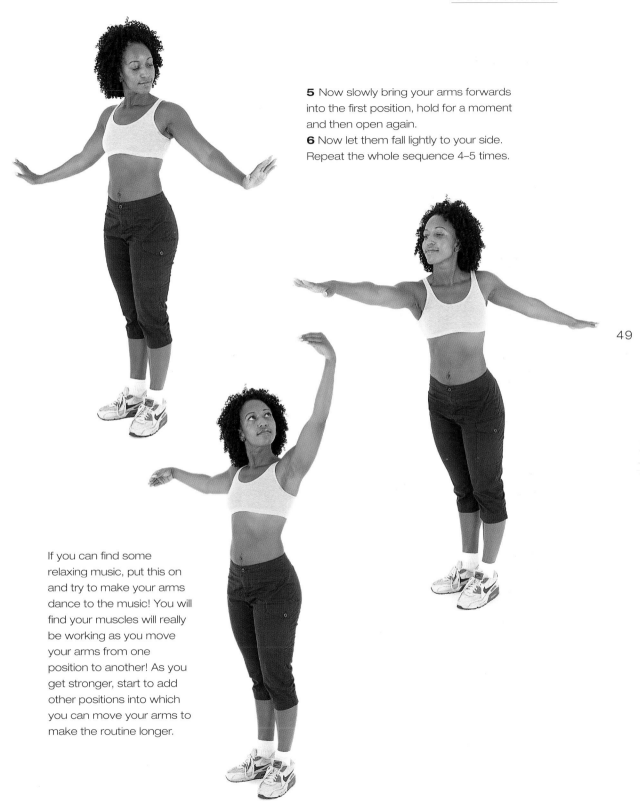

5 Now slowly bring your arms forwards into the first position, hold for a moment and then open again.

6 Now let them fall lightly to your side. Repeat the whole sequence 4–5 times.

If you can find some relaxing music, put this on and try to make your arms dance to the music! You will find your muscles will really be working as you move your arms from one position to another! As you get stronger, start to add other positions into which you can move your arms to make the routine longer.

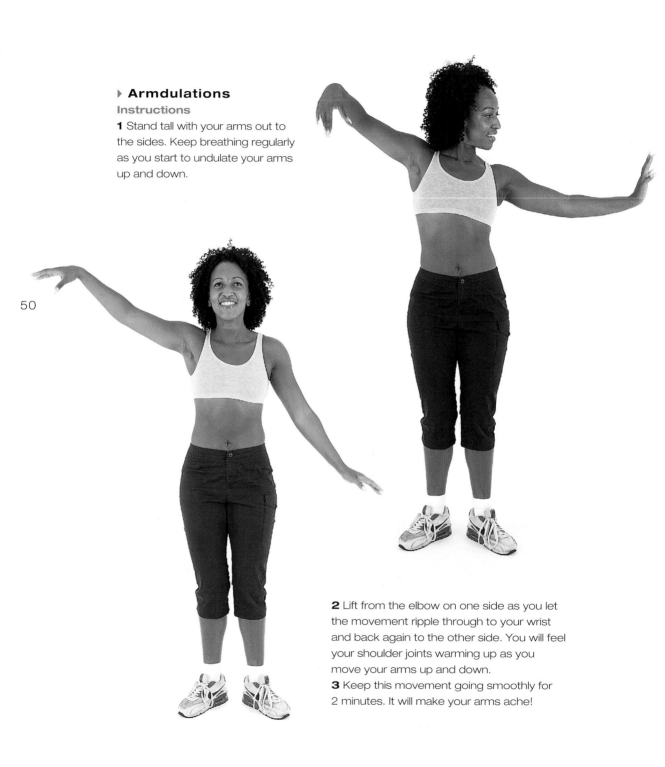

▶ **Armdulations**

Instructions

1 Stand tall with your arms out to the sides. Keep breathing regularly as you start to undulate your arms up and down.

2 Lift from the elbow on one side as you let the movement ripple through to your wrist and back again to the other side. You will feel your shoulder joints warming up as you move your arms up and down.

3 Keep this movement going smoothly for 2 minutes. It will make your arms ache!

▸ Handstand

Another way to perform a static hold is to do a handstand.

Instructions

1 Find a solid wall that you can kick against and then kick your legs up and lean against the wall.
2 As you stay there, pull in on your abdominal muscles to support your weight, and press up through your arms and shoulders. Because all your body weight is bearing down on your arms you will tone up in no time!
3 Hold for 10 breaths if you can. Build up to 20 breaths.

▾ Static hold

Any exercise, such as this, in which you have to support your body weight with your arms will automatically stress and thus tone your arm muscles.

Instructions

1 Adopt the press-up position with your feet tucked underneath you and your back perfectly straight.
2 Hold this position for 20 breaths. Although this exercise works many other muscles besides, your arms are supporting all your weight. This will strengthen and tone them. Release and as you get stronger repeat up to 3 times.

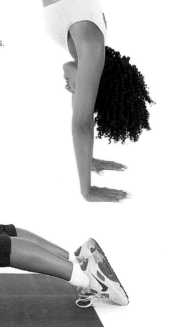

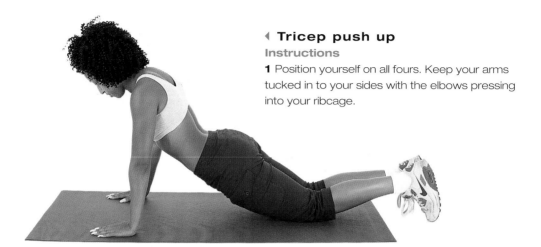

◀ Tricep push up
Instructions

1 Position yourself on all fours. Keep your arms tucked in to your sides with the elbows pressing into your ribcage.

2 Now press your hips forwards as much as you can, whilst keeping your weight forwards over your wrists.

3 Bend your arms so that your whole body lowers towards the floor. Keep the elbows still tucked in next to your ribs. Hold for 1 second and press your arms out straight again. Repeat up to 20 times.

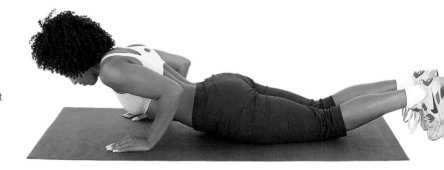

4 Keeping your elbows tucked in focuses the workload on the tricep muscle at the back of the arm. As you get stronger (after six weeks), take the push up into the full prone position, building up to 20 repetitions.

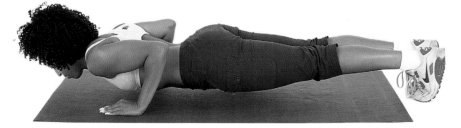

▾ Wide angle press up

Instructions

1 Get down on to your hands and knees, with your feet crossed, and press your hips forwards. Position your arms so that they are a shoulder width and a half apart.

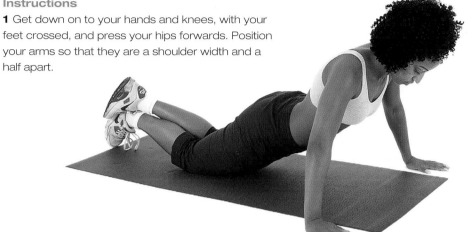

53

2 In this position, bend your arms and lower your body until it is just off the floor. Straighten your arms again. Repeat this exercise up to 20 times. Aim to get low enough so that your arms are at right angles.

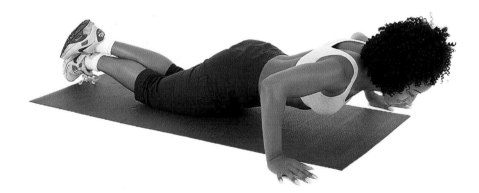

You're toning the chest muscles and triceps muscle in this exercise. As you get stronger, do it in the full push-up position and build up to 25 repetitions.

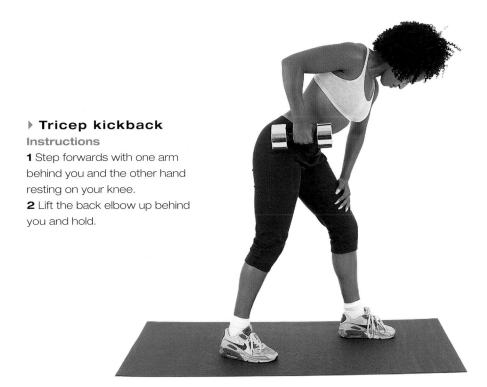

▶ Tricep kickback

Instructions

1 Step forwards with one arm behind you and the other hand resting on your knee.

2 Lift the back elbow up behind you and hold.

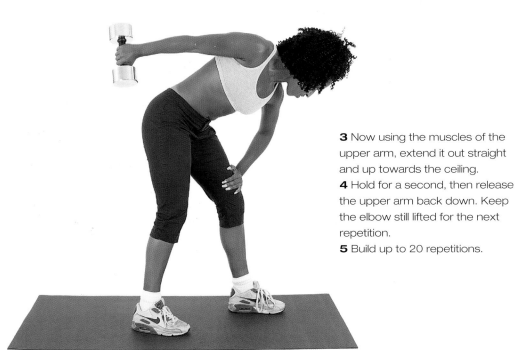

3 Now using the muscles of the upper arm, extend it out straight and up towards the ceiling.

4 Hold for a second, then release the upper arm back down. Keep the elbow still lifted for the next repetition.

5 Build up to 20 repetitions.

▼ Preacher curl with weight

Instructions

1 If you really want to focus on the bicep muscle along the front of the arm, then sit on a chair and, holding a small hand weight, press your upper arm against one thigh.

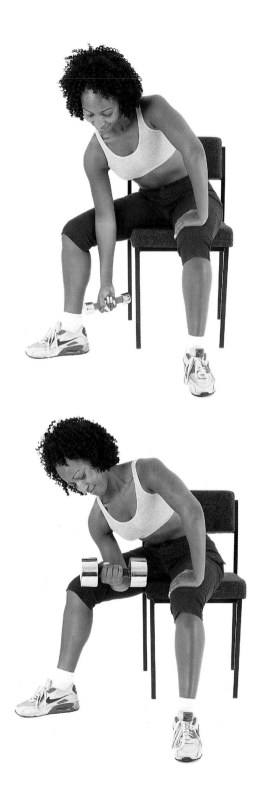

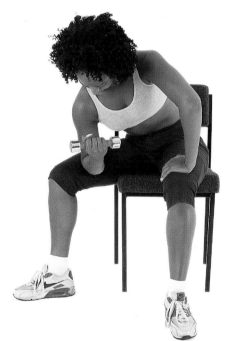

2 Slowly contract the bicep muscle to bend your arm. Hold for a second, then slowly release down again. Repeat 15–20 times and then repeat on the other side.

3 In this position, you can really see the muscle working and therefore you can focus on it and ensure that you are working it fully. As you get stronger, you may need to invest in heavier weights to perform the same exercise, but in this case only do it 8 times.

▼ Tricep extension with weight

Instructions

1 Stand with the correct posture (*see* page 36) and then lift a weight in one hand.

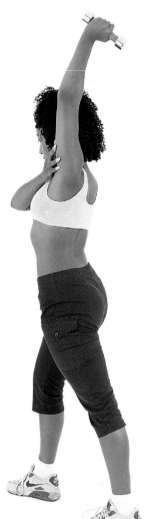

2 Drop the hand holding the weight down behind your back, using your other arm to keep the first in position. Straighten your arm so the end of the weight pushes towards the ceiling. Hold momentarily and bend again.

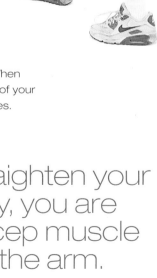

3 As you straighten and bend, make sure that your back is not becoming arched or that the elbow of your working arm is not drifting lower.

4 Aim for 20 repetitions on each arm. When this becomes easy, increase the weight of your dumbbells until you can only lift 8–10 times.

When you straighten your arm in this way, you are utilizing the tricep muscle in the back of the arm.

▼ Tricep extension with weight prone

Instructions

1 Lie on a bench or a bed and hold a weight in both hands and directly above your chest.

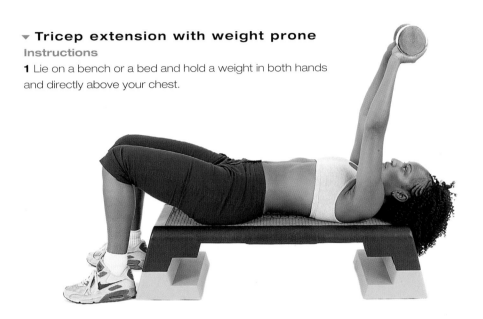

2 Slowly bend your arms to lower the weight back over your head. Control this movement slowly and then straighten your arms again.

3 As you bend and then straighten your arms in this position you are once again focusing on the triceps muscle at the back of the arms.

4 Repeat up to 20 times and, when you get stronger, try increasing the weight gradually until you can only just perform 8–10 repetitions.

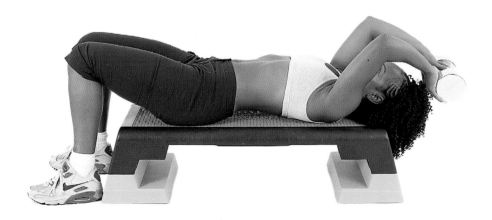

stomach **workout**

The stomach is the prime area that most people want to focus on with the objective of flattening and strengthening it. It is made up of three bands of muscle: the rectus abdominus muscle which runs down the centre of the abdominal area; the internal and external oblique muscles which wrap around the sides of the waist; and the transverse muscle which is the deepest band that runs across the stomach area. In order to tone and shape the abdominal area you will have to work on all these muscles. The exercises that are featured in the following pages show you how to tone all of them.

▼ Basic curl up

The basic curl up is always worth doing to tone the rectus abdominus muscle which runs down the front of the stomach. As you lift your head and shoulders, the rectus abdominals are contracting from both ends (the muscles attach to the breastbone and the pelvis) to lift one end of the body.

Instructions

1 Place your hands on the sides of your head to aid the neck muscles in lifting your head and, as you curl, make sure you lift your shoulder blades off the floor.

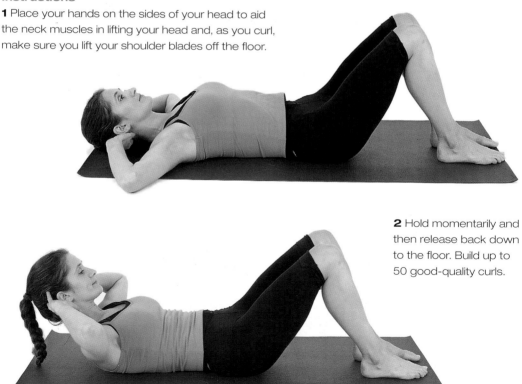

2 Hold momentarily and then release back down to the floor. Build up to 50 good-quality curls.

▼ Pulse curl

Instructions

1 Lie on the floor with your arms by your sides, knees bent and feet flat on the floor. Start curling up, lifting your head and shoulders off the floor and reaching forwards with your arms.

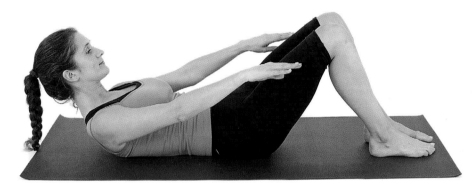

2 Curl up as high as you can, and when you get to this point extend your arms and then lift and lower just an inch or two in this position. This will work the muscles in an intensive way because you are not going through the whole range of movement. Build up to 20 repetitions of the pulse and then lower, rest and repeat.

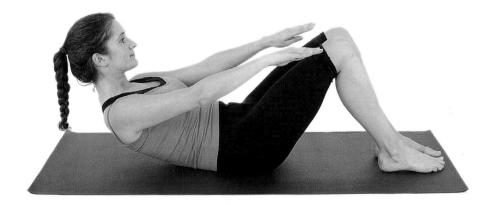

▼ Cross curl

Instructions

1 Adopt the position shown below.

2 Press the thigh of your crossed leg outwards as you wrap your hand around it. Now lift up and across to press your elbow towards your knee and then gently release back down to the floor. Build up gradually to 20 repetitions on each side.

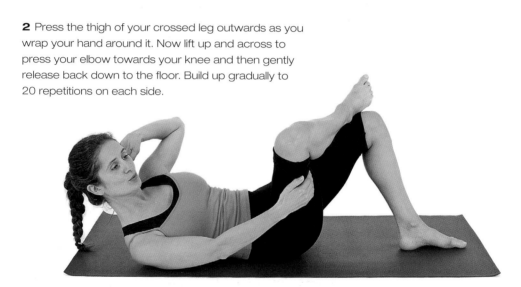

▼ Side reach

Instructions

1 Start by doing a basic curl up position
and hold.

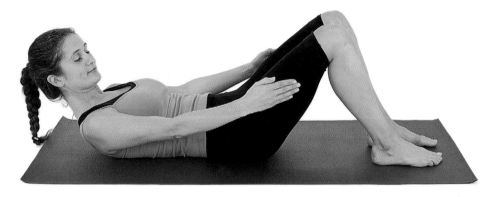

2 Now reach out with one hand towards
your outer calf.

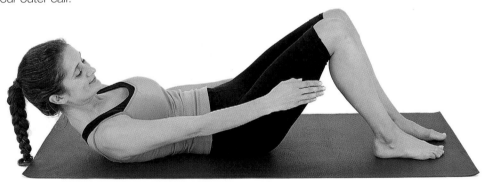

3 Perform 20 pulses reaching down towards your
ankle. With these small movements you are again
focusing on the oblique muscles which wrap
around the sides of the torso. Build up to 50
repetitions (over a period of weeks) on each side.

▼ Tension hold

There are many different ways to perform tension holds. They were originally used by gymnasts to give them perfect body tension for aerial moves. They have now entered the general fitness vocabulary as they strengthen the deep transverse muscles which cross the stomach area.

Instructions

1 Adopt the position shown here (left) and hold for 20–30 seconds

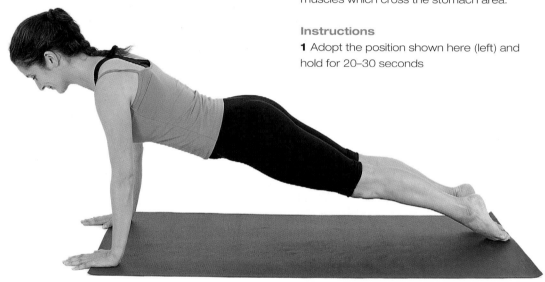

2 As you hold this position, keep breathing regularly and check that your stomach muscles are contracting and working hard to maintain your body in a plank shape. You should not be sagging in the middle; nor should you be sticking your bottom in the air.
3 Rest after 30 seconds and then repeat the exercise once more.

▶ Double leg push out

Instructions

1 Sit with your legs bent, your hands supporting you behind. Your toes should be just touching the floor with your heels lifted off it.

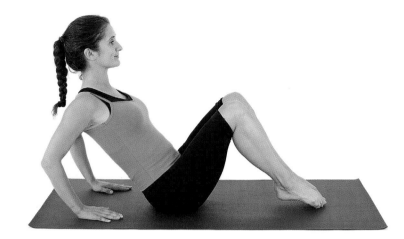

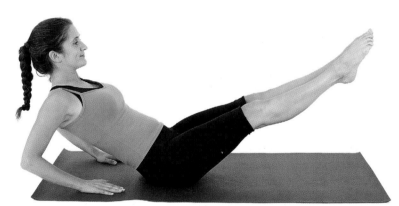

2 Now lean back and shoot your legs out straight in front of you.
3 Bring them back in again. Repeat this up to 20 times. You will feel, and see, the transverse muscles working as you extend your legs.

4 As you become stronger, you can shoot your legs out on the diagonal, first in one direction, then the other and then back to the centre. Build up to 20 of these, too.

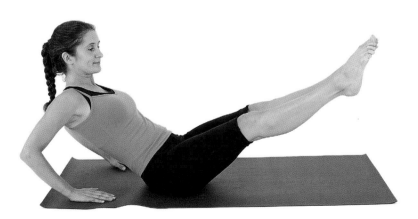
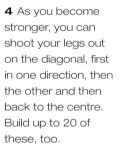

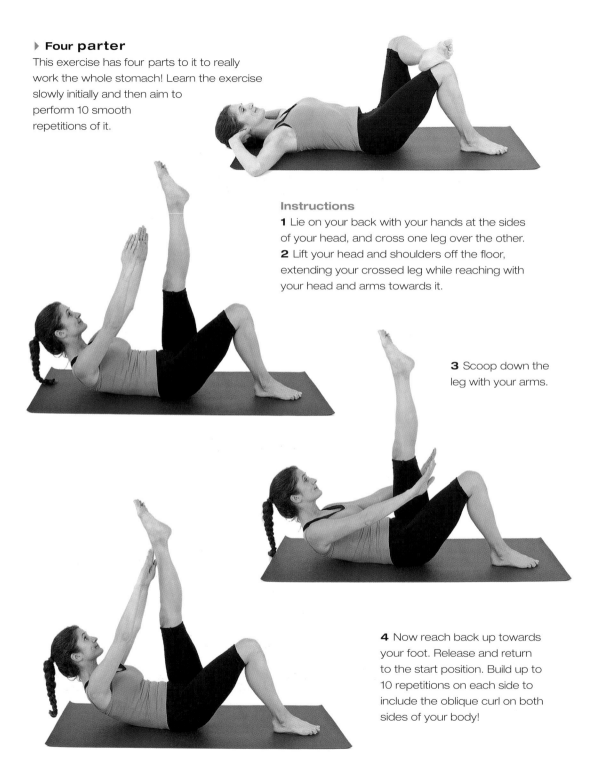

▶ Four parter

This exercise has four parts to it to really work the whole stomach! Learn the exercise slowly initially and then aim to perform 10 smooth repetitions of it.

Instructions

1 Lie on your back with your hands at the sides of your head, and cross one leg over the other.
2 Lift your head and shoulders off the floor, extending your crossed leg while reaching with your head and arms towards it.

3 Scoop down the leg with your arms.

4 Now reach back up towards your foot. Release and return to the start position. Build up to 10 repetitions on each side to include the oblique curl on both sides of your body!

▼ Long arm curl

Instructions

1 Lie back on the floor with your knees bent and stretch both arms out behind your head.

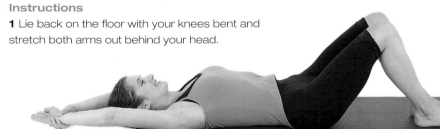

2 Hold one hand with the other and start to lift your head and shoulders off the floor, very gradually. Keep your arms by your ears as you exhale and use your abdominals to lift your upper body off the floor.

65

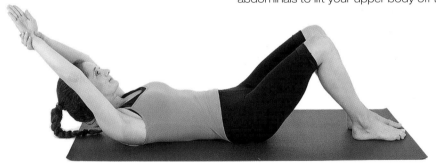

3 Lift first to one level, and then lift a little higher. Hold for a moment, then lower your body down again with control. Build up to 20 controlled repetitions.

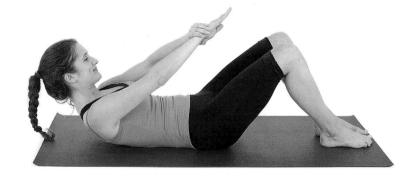

▼ Leg kick ups

Instructions

1 Lie on your back with your hands stretched out behind your head and your legs straight.

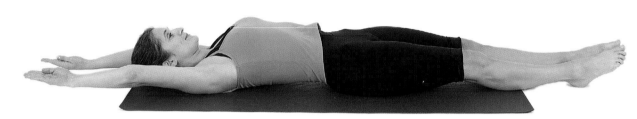

2 Use your stomach strength to bring one leg to meet your arms as you sit up. Release back down to the floor and repeat, bringing the other leg up this time. If you build up a rhythm doing these moves you will find them easier. Try to perform 20 if you can.

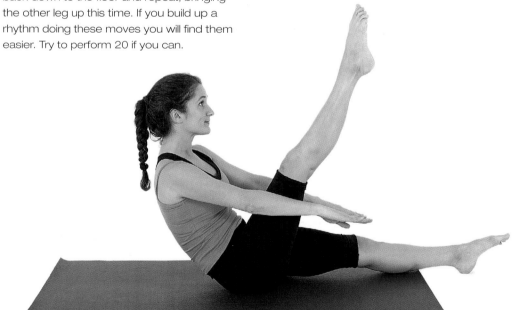

3 This exercise is quite difficult but you can make it easier by keeping the other leg bent and raising both arms as you lift.

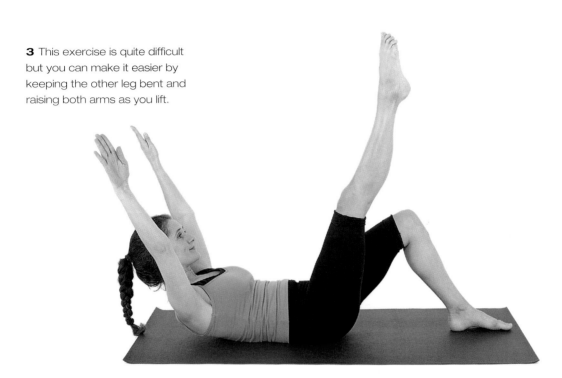

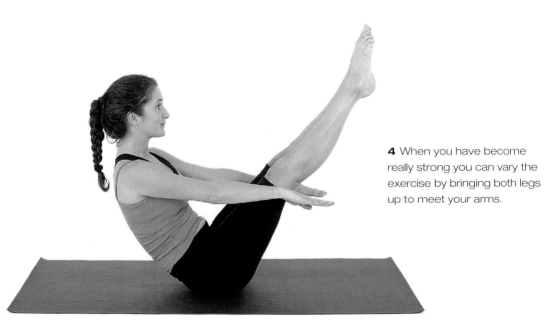

4 When you have become really strong you can vary the exercise by bringing both legs up to meet your arms.

bottom workout

The muscles of the bottom are the gluteus maximus and minimus. Every time you contract your bottom you are using these muscles – so get clenching and tone up this important area!

▼ Butt clencher

Instructions

1 Lie on the floor with your knees bent. Now lift your hips up towards the ceiling. As you do this, focus on squeezing your buttock muscles and use this as the impetus to shoot your hips up.

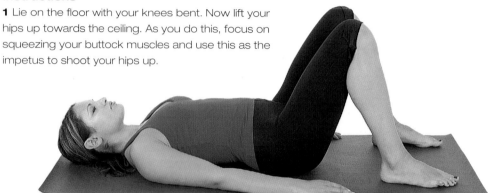

2 Perform 20 of these movements, then rest.
3 Now lift your hips in the same way but stay up at the top and pulse your hips towards the ceiling. Do 20 pulses before you lower.

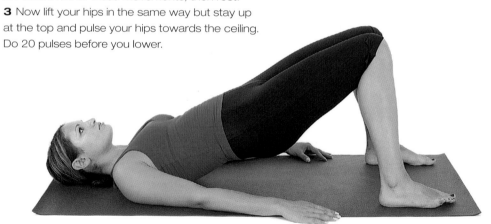

▼ Bridge work

Instructions

1 Lie on your back as before and lift your hips towards the ceiling.

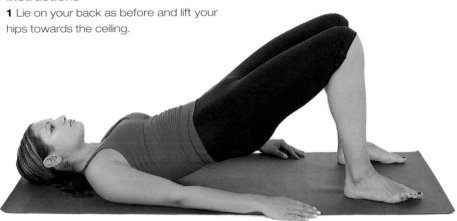

2 Now open and close your knees, using your buttock muscles and inside leg muscles to really squeeze your legs together and then press them open again.
3 Do 20 of these open and close movements before you relax to the floor.

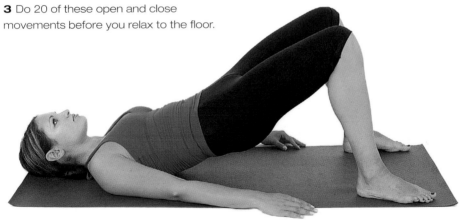

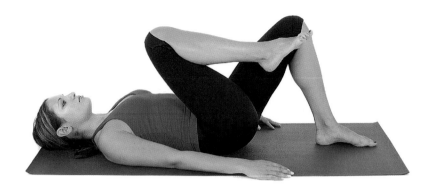

▶ One hip pulse

Instructions

1 Lie on your back, as on page 68, with your knees bent. Start with a series of hip lifts up and down to get you into a rhythm.

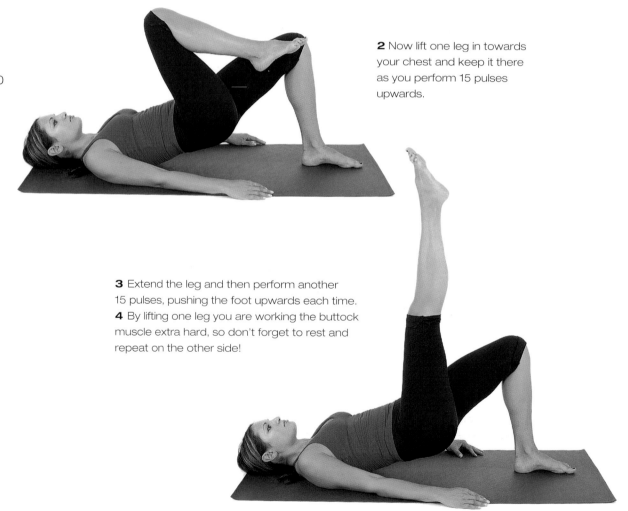

2 Now lift one leg in towards your chest and keep it there as you perform 15 pulses upwards.

3 Extend the leg and then perform another 15 pulses, pushing the foot upwards each time.
4 By lifting one leg you are working the buttock muscle extra hard, so don't forget to rest and repeat on the other side!

▼ Dorsal extenders

Instructions

1 Lie on your stomach with your head resting on your hands. Start by extending one foot along the ground and really lengthening and extending the foot away from you.

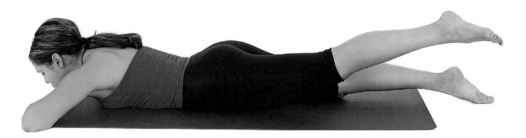

2 Now lift and lower both legs with control. Lift them just a foot or so off the ground and then release to the floor.

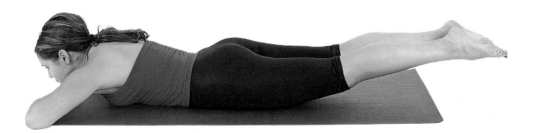

3 Repeat with alternate legs.
4 When you become really strong, you can try lifting both legs off the floor. This will tone your back muscles as well as the buttocks.

▶ Attitude lifts

Instructions

1 Stand holding on to a wall, a barre or the back of a chair. Draw one foot up to the side of your other leg and hold with the ball of your foot pressing against the knee.

2 Now press the bent leg out behind you and hold. As you hold, check the position of the leg: your knee should be higher than your foot, and your hips should be still facing forwards.

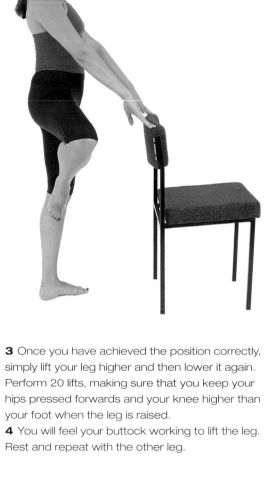

3 Once you have achieved the position correctly, simply lift your leg higher and then lower it again. Perform 20 lifts, making sure that you keep your hips pressed forwards and your knee higher than your foot when the leg is raised.

4 You will feel your buttock working to lift the leg. Rest and repeat with the other leg.

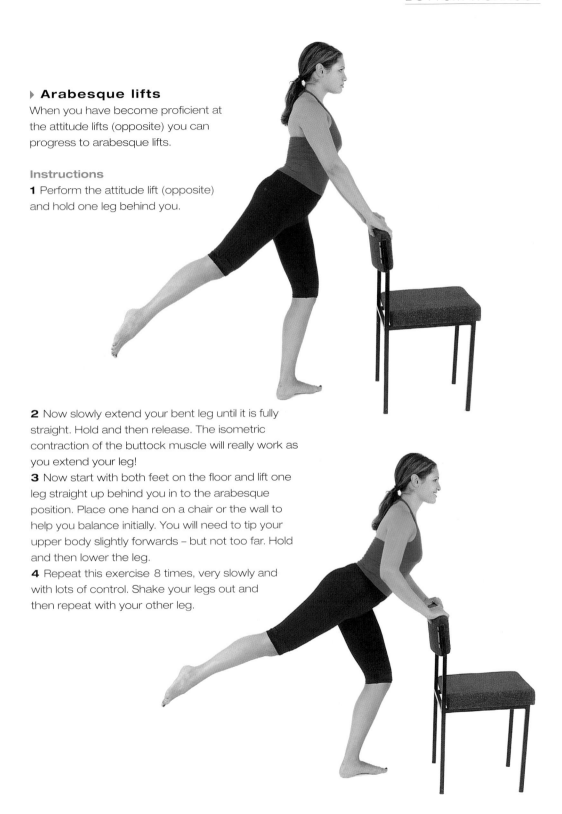

▶ Arabesque lifts

When you have become proficient at
the attitude lifts (opposite) you can
progress to arabesque lifts.

Instructions

1 Perform the attitude lift (opposite)
and hold one leg behind you.

2 Now slowly extend your bent leg until it is fully
straight. Hold and then release. The isometric
contraction of the buttock muscle will really work as
you extend your leg!
3 Now start with both feet on the floor and lift one
leg straight up behind you in to the arabesque
position. Place one hand on a chair or the wall to
help you balance initially. You will need to tip your
upper body slightly forwards – but not too far. Hold
and then lower the leg.
4 Repeat this exercise 8 times, very slowly and
with lots of control. Shake your legs out and
then repeat with your other leg.

▶ All fours fix
Instructions

1 Position yourself on the floor on your hands and knees with your back straight.

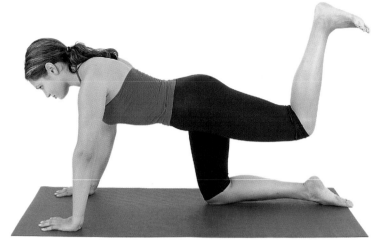

2 Now lift one leg up behind you with your leg bent and your thigh parallel to the floor. Gently lift and lower the thigh about 5 cm (2 in) up and then down again. Perform 15–20 lifts and lowers and then lower the leg back down to the floor.

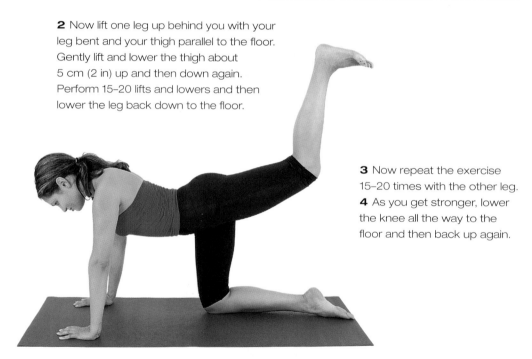

3 Now repeat the exercise 15–20 times with the other leg.
4 As you get stronger, lower the knee all the way to the floor and then back up again.

Don't let your head come up too far or your back may start to arch.

▾ All fours further

Instructions

1 Position yourself on all fours as before. But this time lower your arms until you are resting on your elbows.
2 Now straighten one leg behind you so that the toe just touches the floor. Check that your hips are facing the floor and then tighten your stomach muscles to keep your back straight.

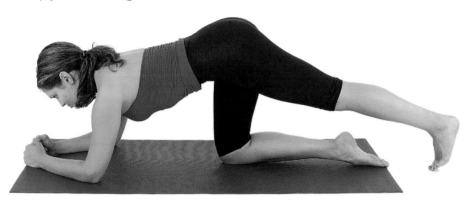

3 Lift your straight leg up as high as you can, without letting your back arch, and then lower it back down again.
4 Perform 15–20 repetitions and then repeat the exercise with the other leg.

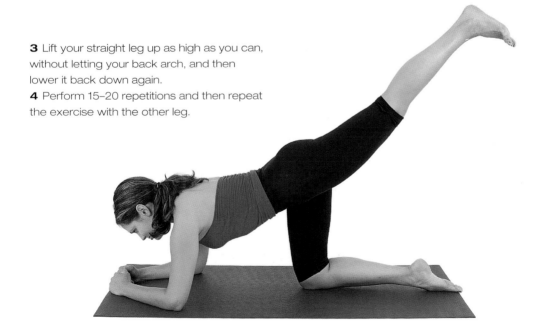

▸ Tuck under tightener

This is a four-part exercise which will tone your thighs and bottom!

Instructions

1 Stand with your legs apart and your hands resting on the back of a chair to help you balance.
2 Turn your feet out, just slightly, and then press your knees out, very slowly, so that you lower into a plie.
3 You should feel this in the back of your thighs and your bottom.

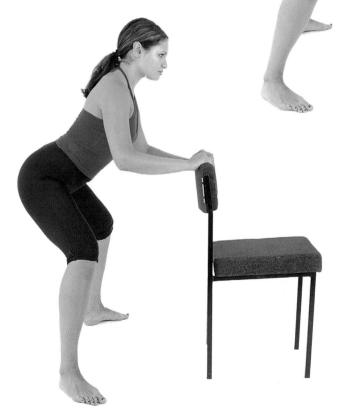

4 Now tilt your backside behind.

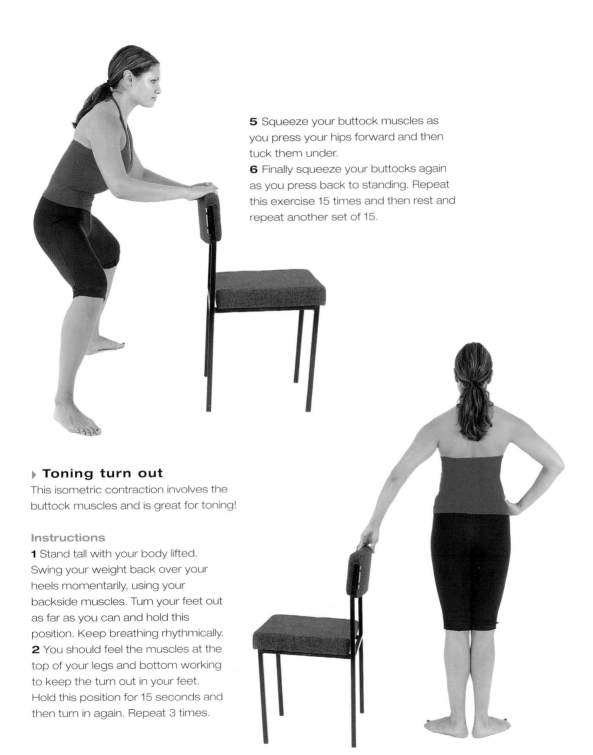

5 Squeeze your buttock muscles as you press your hips forward and then tuck them under.

6 Finally squeeze your buttocks again as you press back to standing. Repeat this exercise 15 times and then rest and repeat another set of 15.

▶ Toning turn out

This isometric contraction involves the buttock muscles and is great for toning!

Instructions

1 Stand tall with your body lifted. Swing your weight back over your heels momentarily, using your backside muscles. Turn your feet out as far as you can and hold this position. Keep breathing rhythmically.

2 You should feel the muscles at the top of your legs and bottom working to keep the turn out in your feet. Hold this position for 15 seconds and then turn in again. Repeat 3 times.

hip and thigh workout

This section of the workout programme is dedicated to working and toning your hips and thighs. The exercises on these pages work the all-important hip area muscles.

▶ Corner lift

Instructions

1 Position yourself on all-fours with your back straight. Pull in on the stomach muscles to support your back.

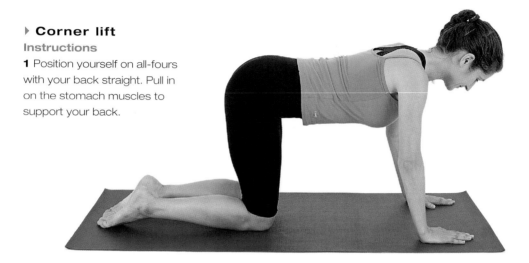

2 Now lift one leg, bent out to the side, and hold. Then slowly lower it. As you lift your leg out to the side you will feel the muscles at the side of the leg and hip working to lift the leg.

3 Rest and repeat on the other leg. Build up to 15 repetitions on each leg.

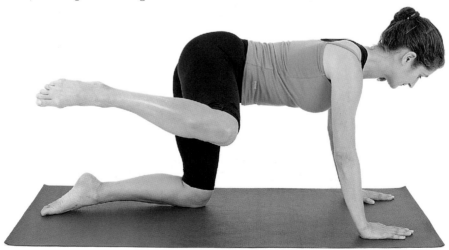

◀ **Leg circles**

Instructions

1 Position yourself as before and then lift your leg out to the side as shown. Hold in this position for a moment and then imagine you have a partner who has lifted their leg opposite you. Now start to circle your leg around the imaginary foot of your partner, first one way and then the other.

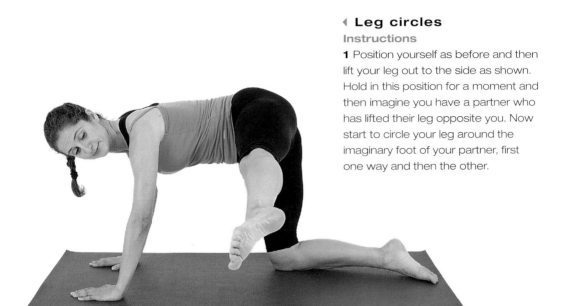

2 This exercise will really make your hips ache! But try and build up to 8 repetitions on each leg.

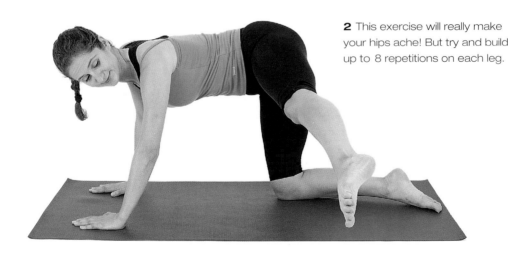

◀ Leg extension

This exercise focuses on the thigh muscles. If wished, you can start off without the leg weights, but wear them as you get stronger to increase the intensity of the exercise.

Instructions

1 Sit on a chair with a straight back, your stomach pulled in and wearing leg weights.

2 Now raise and straighten one leg, hold and release. Repeat this straightening of the leg 20 times. Then repeat on the other leg.

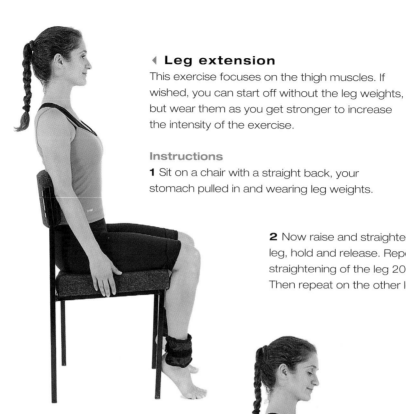

3 As you straighten the leg, focus on the quadriceps muscles on the front of the thigh. These are the muscles that are doing all the work.

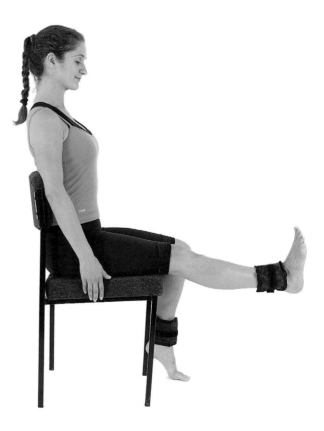

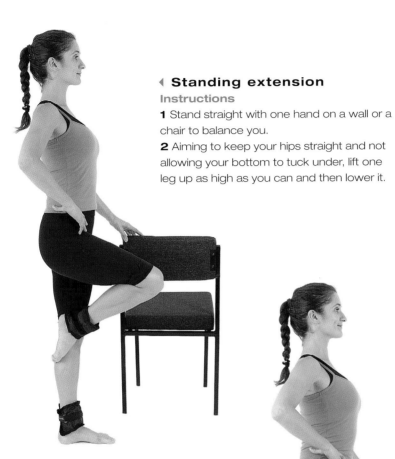

◀ Standing extension

Instructions

1 Stand straight with one hand on a wall or a chair to balance you.

2 Aiming to keep your hips straight and not allowing your bottom to tuck under, lift one leg up as high as you can and then lower it.

3 Repeat with the other leg. You are using the quadriceps muscles and the hip flexors at the front of the body in this exercise.

4 As you become stronger and more flexible, you can start to swing the leg a little more, but make sure you control it on the way down.

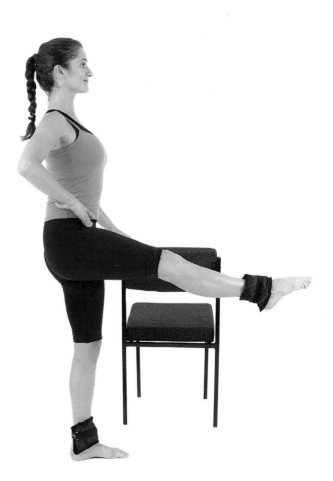

▼ Side lying extension

1 Lie on the floor on one side and prop yourself up on your elbows. Straighten your legs on the floor but extend your feet and pull up on your knees to lengthen your legs.

2 Now, with your upper leg raised, bend the knee. Extend your raised leg slowly, pointing your toes.

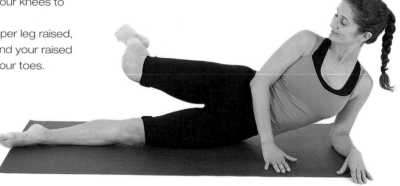

82

3 Bend your leg and extend it again quickly, then slowly lower the leg down to the floor. Repeat the exercise up to 8 times.

4 Now turn over and repeat the exercise up to 8 times on the other side.

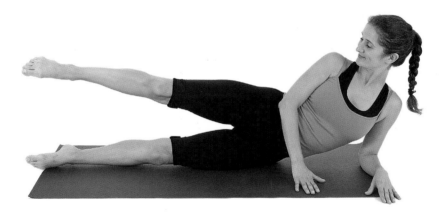

As you bend and straighten the leg, perform each move slowly. It should feel as though you are moving your leg through syrup.

▶ Side lying leg lift

Do not tip the hips back so that the leg goes up all the way – if this happens, you will not be using the abductor muscles at the side of the thigh.

Instructions

1 Lie on your side with your arm propping you up. Make sure that you keep your neck extended and your stomach muscles tight. Tip your hips slightly forwards so that your other hand is resting on the floor in front of you.

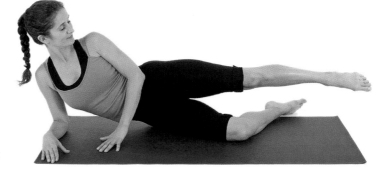

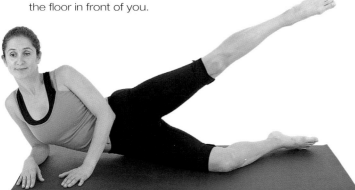

2 Now, with your lower leg bent slightly inwards, extend the foot of your top leg and, with the leg tensed, lift it as high as you can. If you are in the correct position, your leg will only lift to 45 degrees (not 90 degrees).

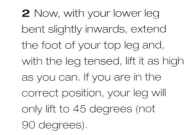

83

3 Hold the lift momentarily and then loweryour leg. Repeat the lift 20 times on each leg.

4 If wished, you can use an alternative arm position for this exercise. Lie on your side as before but prop yourself up on your elbow with your head resting on your hand. Repeat as above.

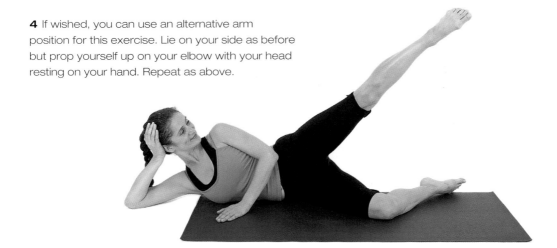

▸ Round the corner toner

Instructions

1 Lie on your side with both legs bent, one on top of the other at right angles to your body.

2 Now lift the top leg, keeping your shin facing forwards and so you feel the side of the top thigh working.

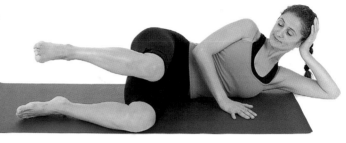

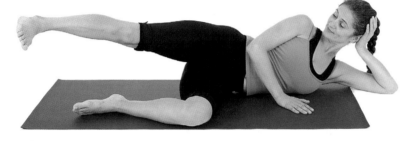

3 Extend your leg until it is straight and hold for a moment.

4 Now bend the leg back to the right angle and lower. Repeat on both legs up to 15 times.

5 As you get stronger, when you straighten the leg swing it round in front of you and then back again for the bend.

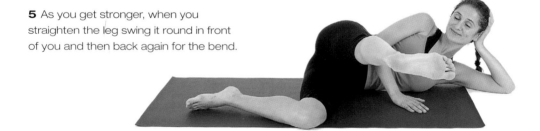

6 To add a further move to this sequence, when the straight leg reaches the front, hold it there and perform 10 pulses in that position before you carry on with the rest of the sequence.

7 You will really feel it in the side of your thighs! Don't forget to do this whole sequence equally on both legs.

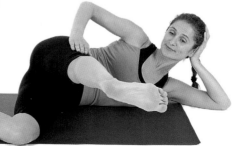

▼ Tap and tip

Instructions

1 Lie on your side, as for the exercise opposite, with one knee bent.
2 Extend the other leg out in front of you. Using your hand to steady you, lift the straight leg all the way up (so that it is parallel with the wall behind) and then lower it to the floor again.

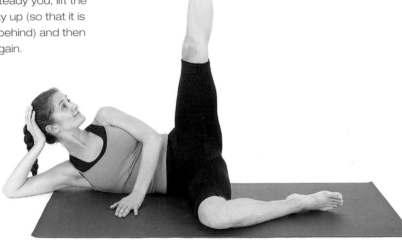

3 Tap your foot lightly on the floor and lift your leg back up again. Perform this tap and lift 10 times on each leg. Keep your abdominals pulled in to support your spine and keep breathing rhythmically.

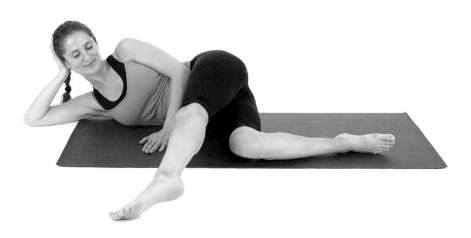

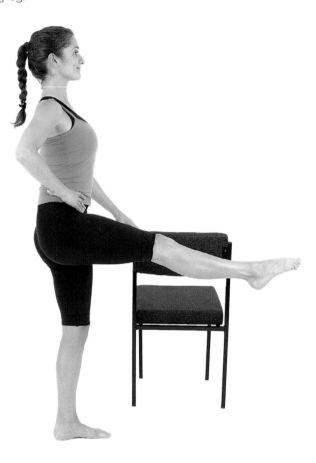

▼ Three way toner

Instructions

1 Stand with one arm against a wall or chair to balance you and then turn out the knee of your raised leg as you draw up your foot to the knee of the supporting leg.

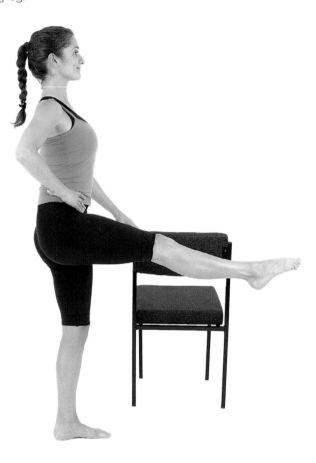

To really tone and shape your thighs, try the ballerina's favourite exercise as shown here.

2 Now very slowly extend the lifted bent leg until it is straight in front of you and hold. Check that you are not letting your hips pull underneath you and that you are lifting up and out through the top of the head as much as you can.

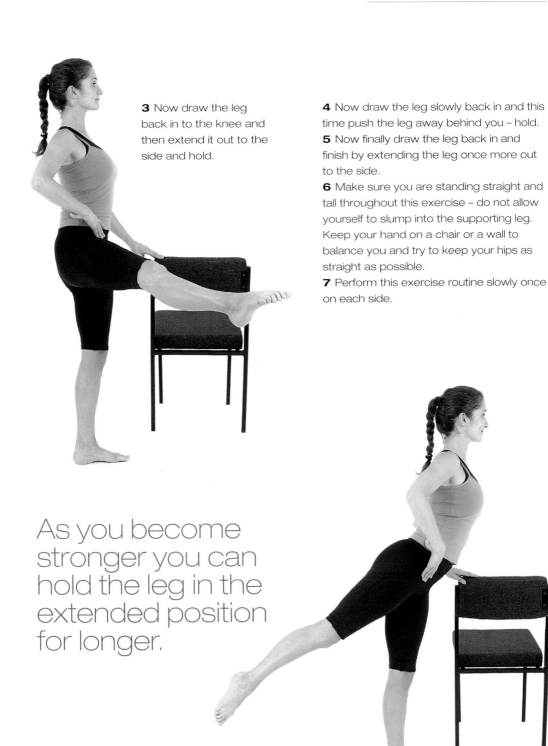

3 Now draw the leg back in to the knee and then extend it out to the side and hold.

4 Now draw the leg slowly back in and this time push the leg away behind you – hold.
5 Now finally draw the leg back in and finish by extending the leg once more out to the side.
6 Make sure you are standing straight and tall throughout this exercise – do not allow yourself to slump into the supporting leg. Keep your hand on a chair or a wall to balance you and try to keep your hips as straight as possible.
7 Perform this exercise routine slowly once on each side.

As you become stronger you can hold the leg in the extended position for longer.

back and shoulder
workout

The shoulders and back are important areas to keep strong. Toning the deltoid muscles of your shoulders will give you strength and a good shape on the top half of your body. Strengthening your back will help keep your posture correct and ward off any back problems.

▶ Shoulder press

1 Stand with your arms by your side and correct posture (*see* page 36). Hold a dumbbell in each hand. Now bend your arms so that the weights are resting just above your shoulders.

2 Press your arms straight into the air, hold and lower. When you straighten your arms do not slam them straight and lock out the elbows. Keep the lock off your elbows.

3 As you do this exercise, focus on your shoulder muscles, which are doing the work. Aim to build up to 25 repetitions of this and you will really feel the deltoid (shoulder) muscles working.

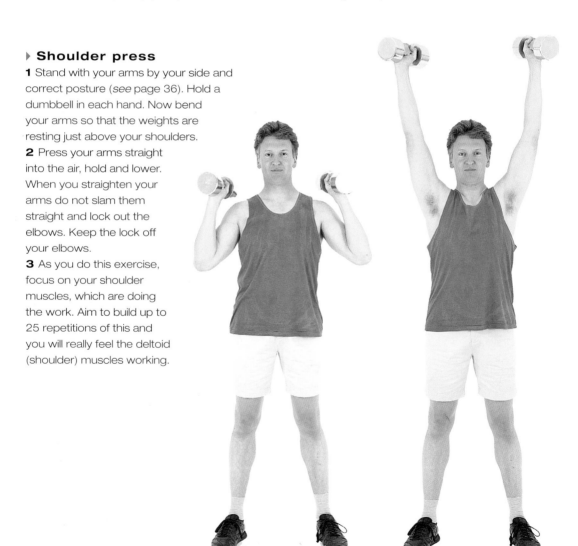

▼ Front deltoid lift

Instructions

1 Stand holding the dumbbells and pull up on the abdominals. Lift one arm slowly out in front of you until your hand reaches chest height.

2 Hold for a moment and then lower slowly. The deltoid muscles (particularly the anterior portion) are doing the major work here. Now lift your other arm in the same way and lower again. Build up to 25 repetitions on each arm.

3 To make this exercise tougher, you can do 25 repetitions first on one arm and then on the other, thereby tiring one set of muscles before moving on to the next.

4 To really push the endurance even further, try doing 10–15 repetitions of lifting both arms together. However, be sure to keep your posture absolutely correct as you do this and try not to lean backwards.

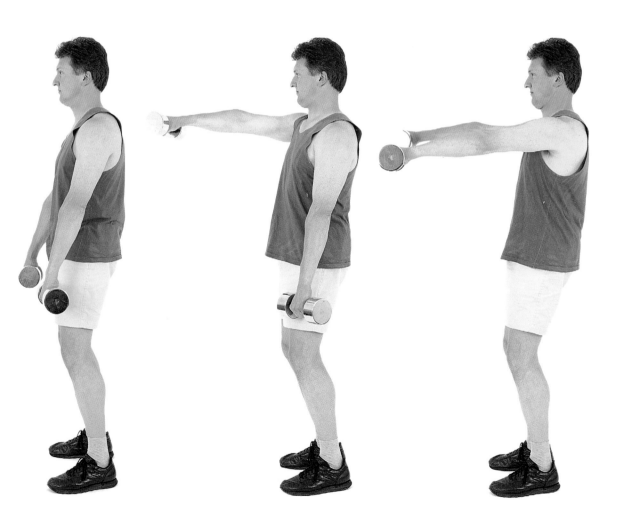

▼ Inverted push up

This exercise works the shoulder muscles by transferring your body weight onto your arms.

Instructions

1 Rest on your hands and feet to begin this exercise but push your backside high up in the air. You will feel your weight on your hands and shoulders and on the balls of your feet.

2 Now begin to bend your arms so that your head is aiming towards the floor. Bend just a few inches and then push your arms until they are straight again.

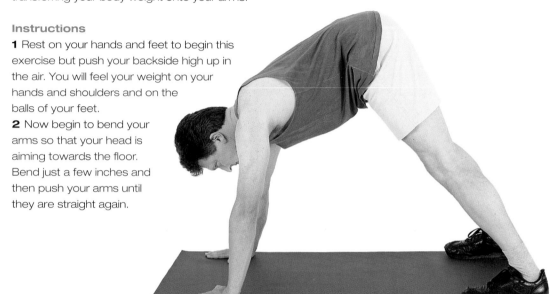

3 The further you lean your weight over your arms, the more you will use your shoulders to push away as you straighten.

4 Be careful in this exercise not to lose control and build up very gradually. Start with 5–8 repetitions for the first 6 weeks, then build up to 15 if you can.

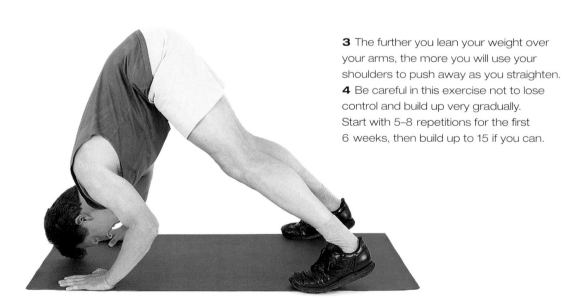

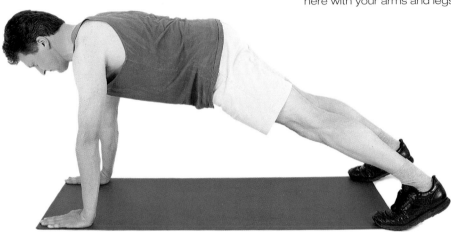

▼ Downward dips

Instructions

1 Place yourself in the position shown here with your arms and legs straight.

2 Breathe deeply for 5 breaths and then start to transfer your weight slightly forwards on to your hands as you lift your head.
3 Now with a more percussive movement, push back with your arms and shoulders so that you shoot your backside to the ceiling. Hold momentarily and then lower. Repeat the exercise up to 20 times.
4 As you push with your arms you will be building up your shoulder (and arm) strength.

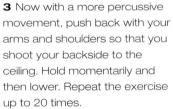
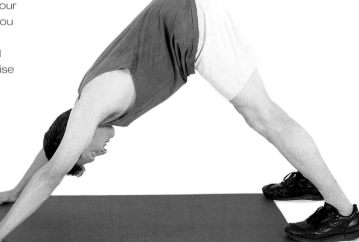

▼ Hyperextension

This exercise is a classic back strengthener and there are many variations and levels of working. It strengthens the erector spinae muscles along either side of the spine which, along with the abdominal muscles, help to move and support the torso.

Instructions

1 Start by lying on your stomach with your hands crossed on the small of your back.

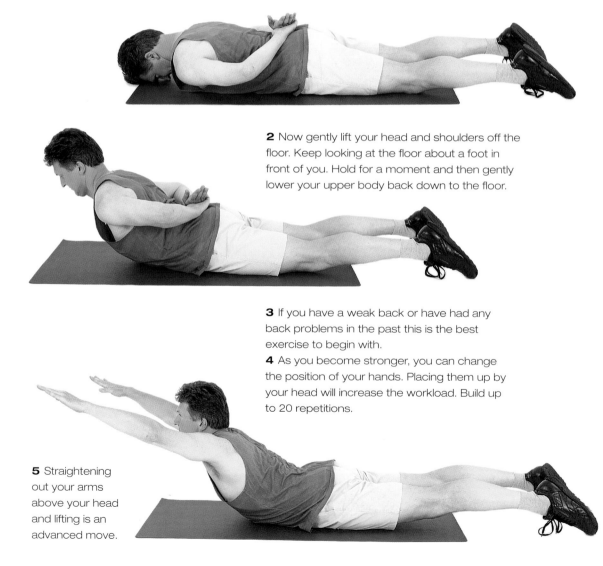

2 Now gently lift your head and shoulders off the floor. Keep looking at the floor about a foot in front of you. Hold for a moment and then gently lower your upper body back down to the floor.

3 If you have a weak back or have had any back problems in the past this is the best exercise to begin with.

4 As you become stronger, you can change the position of your hands. Placing them up by your head will increase the workload. Build up to 20 repetitions.

5 Straightening out your arms above your head and lifting is an advanced move.

▼ Hyper rock

Once you have mastered the exercise opposite you can make it even tougher by lifting your legs at the same time so that your body is in an arc.

Instructions

1 You are now using your buttock and hamstring muscles as well as your back muscles.

2 Hold this position for several breaths to become comfortable in it.

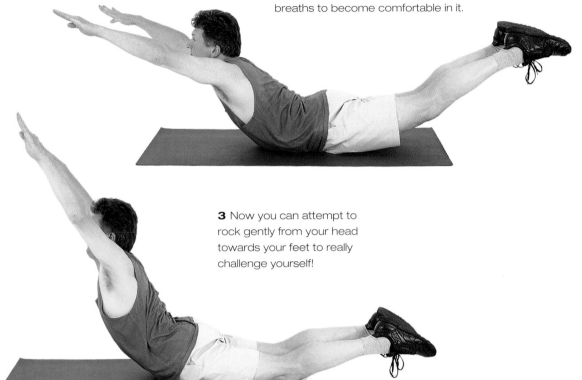

3 Now you can attempt to rock gently from your head towards your feet to really challenge yourself!

4 Perform 5 rocks and then rest and repeat.

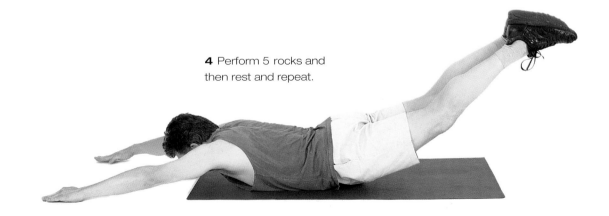

Working on the shoulders, you will need your weights again.

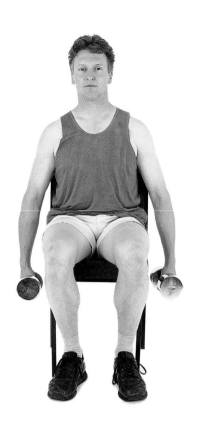

◀ **Seated lat lift**

Instructions

1 Sit straight on a solid chair with a weight in each hand. Now pull in the abdominal muscles and lean slightly forwards for the starting position.

2 Keeping the lock off your elbows, smoothly lift both arms out to the side. Hold and lower them with control.

3 As you control the lowering of the weights you are using the latissimus dorsi muscles in the sides of your back. As you lift the weights, you are using your shoulder muscles, too. Repeat this exercise 10–12 times.

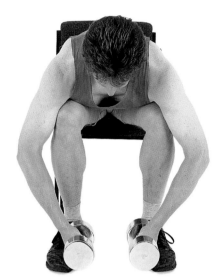

▸ Seated derriere delt

Instructions

1 Sit as before on a solid seat with a weight in each hand and tilt forwards, with a straight back, so that your torso is supported on your legs.

95

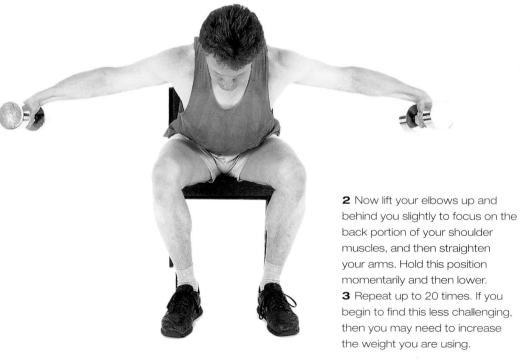

2 Now lift your elbows up and behind you slightly to focus on the back portion of your shoulder muscles, and then straighten your arms. Hold this position momentarily and then lower.

3 Repeat up to 20 times. If you begin to find this less challenging, then you may need to increase the weight you are using.

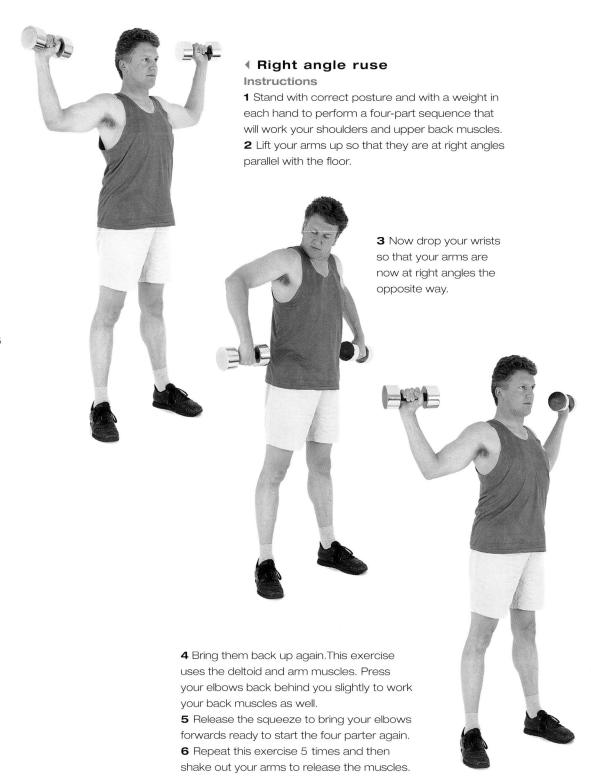

◀ Right angle ruse

Instructions

1 Stand with correct posture and with a weight in each hand to perform a four-part sequence that will work your shoulders and upper back muscles.
2 Lift your arms up so that they are at right angles parallel with the floor.

3 Now drop your wrists so that your arms are now at right angles the opposite way.

4 Bring them back up again. This exercise uses the deltoid and arm muscles. Press your elbows back behind you slightly to work your back muscles as well.
5 Release the squeeze to bring your elbows forwards ready to start the four parter again.
6 Repeat this exercise 5 times and then shake out your arms to release the muscles.

▶ **Diagonal dare**
Instructions

1 Rest on all fours on the floor with your abdominals pulled up to keep your back straight.

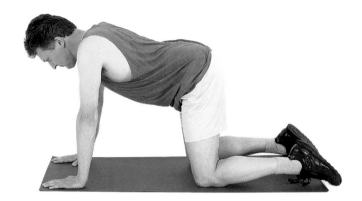

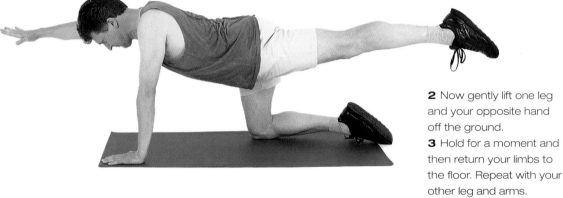

2 Now gently lift one leg and your opposite hand off the ground.

3 Hold for a moment and then return your limbs to the floor. Repeat with your other leg and arms.

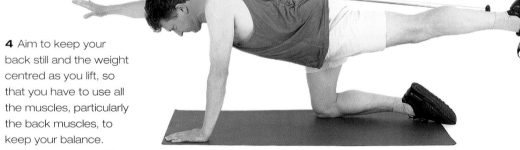

4 Aim to keep your back still and the weight centred as you lift, so that you have to use all the muscles, particularly the back muscles, to keep your balance.

5 Do 10 slow repetitions of this exercise.

6 When you need a new challenge, try to find someone who will place a stick (broom handle) across your back and then perform the same exercise without letting the stick move or fall!

cardiovascular workout

Don't forget that as well as the toning exercises you have been doing, it is important to work the heart and lungs. The heart is a muscle like all other muscles in your body and therefore responds to being challenged by becoming larger and stronger. With your heart and lungs working more efficiently, you will have more energy and vitality than ever before!

▶ Walking

Fast-paced walking is one of the best ways to get your heart going and your blood circulating. It is an activity that can be enjoyed by the majority of people with a smaller risk of injury. Walking can be as light or as challenging as you wish, so within 10 minutes you can play around a little!

Start by walking at a natural pace, looking around you and breathing naturally to give yourself a gentle warm up. Once you have become warmer, you can start to push the pace a little. Walk faster and lengthen your pace so that you are covering more distance with each step.

As you walk in this way, you will feel your breathing become heavier to give you more oxygen as you work harder. Aim to keep this kind of pace up for the full 10 minutes. Afterwards you can do some of the stretches featured in the stretch section as you cool down.

Walking variations

When you have established your walking route you can start introducing some added elements to increase the intensity of your workout.

1 Walk the same distance but faster, thereby speeding up your pace even more. (Don't be tempted to run though.)

2 Walk the same distance but with less steps (you will need to have counted them first!), thereby increasing the length of your strides.

3 Carry some weighted arm bands as you walk.

4 Try changing your pace to the very smallest steps you can. You will really feel this in your calves and ankles.

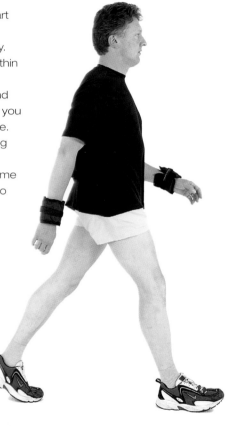

▶ Skipping 10

As your CV sections are only 10 minutes (normally a CV routine aimed at weight loss might take you 20–30 minutes), you can really try to push your heart rate up and then bring it down again. This will give your heart a good workout and allow you to recover, too! Skipping is a great CV routine to do as it will work you hard but you can vary the pace to suit yourself.

Instructions

1 Start by practising your skipping stance. Keep your elbows in at your sides and flick your wrists as if you are holding a rope. Go through the balls of your feet to the heels as you skip from one foot to the other. Keep your feet just off the ground as you transfer your weight.
2 Now try the same thing with the rope. Don't worry if you trip on the rope from time to time – practice will make this happen less and less!

99

Variations:

● Lift one knee as you skip.
● Skip forwards and back and then from side to side.
● Try a star jump move in between the fall of the rope.
● Do a high jump over the rope.
● Skip over the rope with both feet.
● Skip slalom-style, pressing your backside out behind you to one side.

▼ Jogging 10

Fast walking and running are great ways to work your heart and lungs. Running puts most people off because they tend to start off too fast and then get out of breath too quickly! Start your workout with some fast walking. Step out long and fast and swing your arms vigorously by your sides.

When you feel ready, try increasing the fast walking so that it becomes a gentle jog. When you jog (as when you run), strike the ground with the heel first; rolling through your foot for good cushioning. Keep your abdominals tightened to support your back and look around you as you jog. You should be breathing comfortably but heavily.

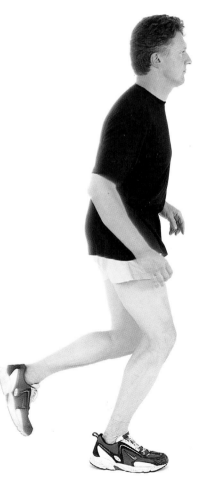

Instructions

1 Start off by jogging for 3 minutes one way, then turn around and jog back for 3 minutes. Finish off with some stretches. Eventually you can build up to 5 minutes' jog one way and 5 minutes back to make the full 10-minute jog.
2 Now add some new challenges to your 10 and skip sideways for 20 seconds.

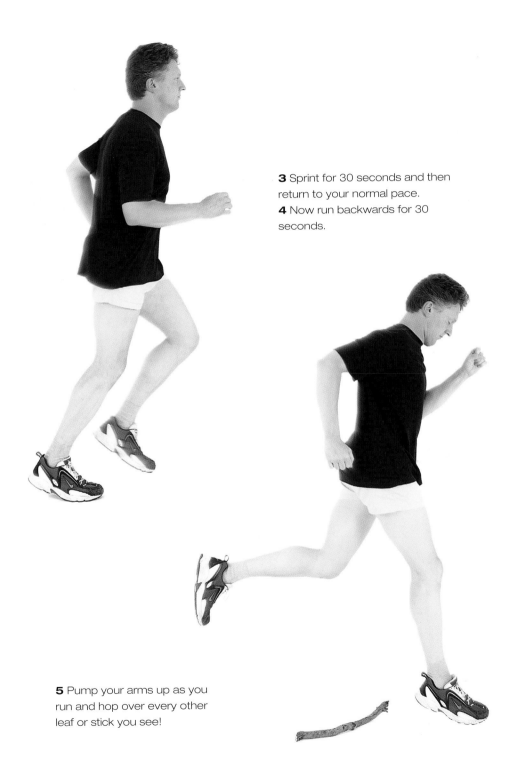

3 Sprint for 30 seconds and then return to your normal pace.
4 Now run backwards for 30 seconds.

5 Pump your arms up as you run and hop over every other leaf or stick you see!

▼ Stepping

You can buy a basic fitness step from most good sports stores. If you cannot get hold of one, you can adapt this routine to fit your flight of stairs or some steps in the park or near your home. Stepping up and down really pushes the heart rate up. You will have noticed this when you climb a steep flight of stairs. So it's a great exercise for you to turn into a 10-minute CV workout.

Instructions

1 Start off by stepping up and down rhythmically on a step to familiarize yourself with the equipment.

2 As you step make sure your whole foot is planted on the step with the heel hitting first. Check your posture as you step; make sure the abdominals are tightened and your shoulders are back and relaxed.

3 Putting on some rhythmical music will help you to step up and down at a regular pace.

4 Aim to keep stepping for the entire 10 minutes. If you find yourself getting really tired, then march on the spot for a couple of minutes to recover and then begin stepping again.

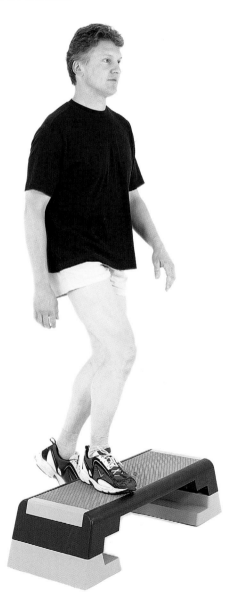

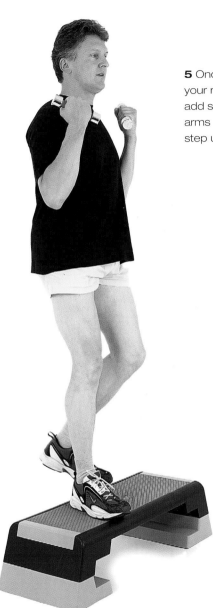

5 Once you have established your rhythm, you can start to add some variations: bend your arms into a bicep curl as you step up and down.

6 Lift one knee and then step back to the floor with each step.
7 Step wide on to the step and narrower on the way back down.
8 To really get your breathing going, jump on to the step and step back down again.

▼ Jumping 10

One of the most natural activities we do as children is to jump. In later life this activity suddenly gets forgotten or is deemed inappropriate but it's a great way to tone muscles and recapture the vitality of life!

First you need to learn how to jump correctly. When you land from a jump, you must go through your toes into the metatarsals and roll through your whole foot. Bend your knees to land safely and protect them and your ankles.

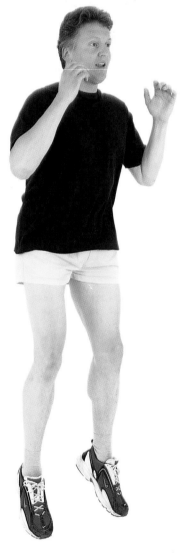

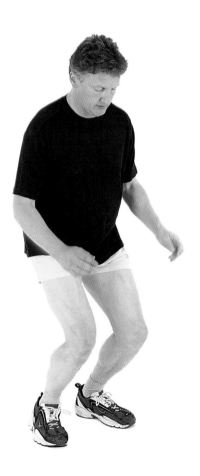

Try some of these jumps and, as you get tired, intersperse them with some jogging on the spot to get your breath back! Aim to do 10–12 of each jump, but take your time. Ensure your technique is good and that you land softly on the ground. This will probably take you 10 minutes with time for some breathers!

Straight jumps

Perform a straight jump with your arms in the air and body straight. Make sure you bend your knees as you land

105

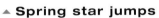

▲ Spring star jumps

Try jumping from and landing in a wide stance, still bending your knees softly into a wide plie as you land.

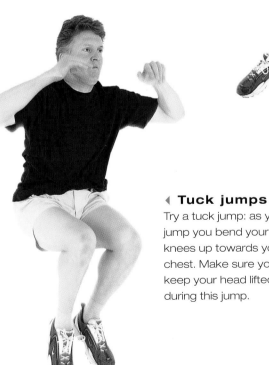

◄ Tuck jumps

Try a tuck jump: as you jump you bend your knees up towards your chest. Make sure you keep your head lifted during this jump.

Small jumps

Turn your feet out slightly, ensuring your knees are in line with your toes. Perform 8–10 small jumps where you leave the ground just high enough to stretch your feet.

top to toe stretch

Now that you have done some toning work you need to ensure you do some sessions on returning your muscles to their proper length. This is where stretching comes in. Every other day, it's a good idea to do a stretching session just to keep your muscles lengthened, your joints fluid and your body supple. This will not only help to prevent injury but it will also give you greater flexibility in your movements.

▸ Extension pose

Instructions

1 Stand up straight, feet hip distance apart, and reach up to the ceiling with both arms.

2 Try to extend your whole body. Lift up from your hips, up through the ribs, and feel yourself growing taller.

3 Now relax into a normal stance and prepare for your Stretch 10.

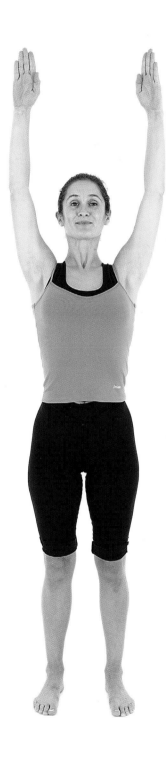

These are passive stretches where you adopt the position and hold for a number of seconds to allow the muscles to lengthen. When you release from a stretch, come out of it slowly and with control.

▸ Neck arc

We often hold a lot of tension in this area so make sure you stretch the muscles in your neck and upper back.

Instructions

1 Stand with your fingers linked over the top of your head.
2 Now gently pull your head forwards and then hold for 10 seconds.
3 Make sure that you keep your stomach pulled in and up and your spine straight so that you are bending only from the neck and the top of your shoulders. This will stretch out your neck muscles and release any tension in your shoulders.

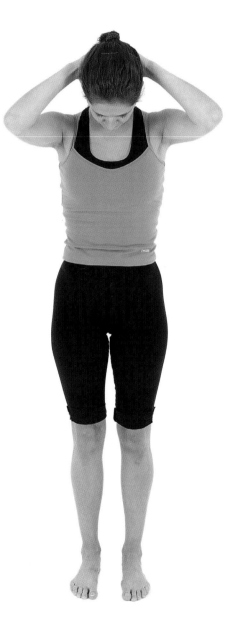

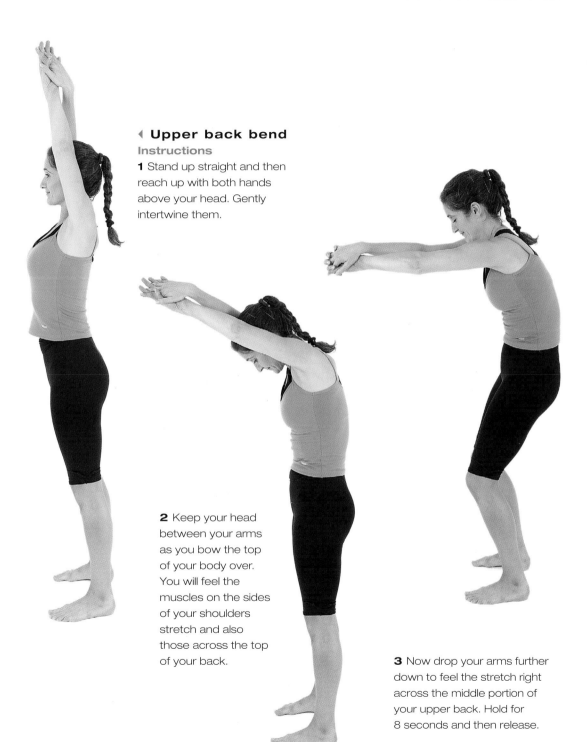

◂ **Upper back bend**

Instructions

1 Stand up straight and then reach up with both hands above your head. Gently intertwine them.

2 Keep your head between your arms as you bow the top of your body over. You will feel the muscles on the sides of your shoulders stretch and also those across the top of your back.

3 Now drop your arms further down to feel the stretch right across the middle portion of your upper back. Hold for 8 seconds and then release.

After working hard on your arms, stretch out the muscles to keep flexible in this area.

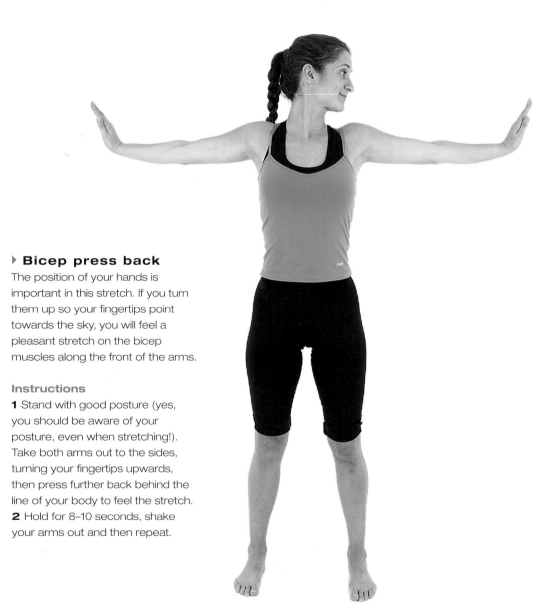

▶ Bicep press back

The position of your hands is important in this stretch. If you turn them up so your fingertips point towards the sky, you will feel a pleasant stretch on the bicep muscles along the front of the arms.

Instructions

1 Stand with good posture (yes, you should be aware of your posture, even when stretching!). Take both arms out to the sides, turning your fingertips upwards, then press further back behind the line of your body to feel the stretch.
2 Hold for 8–10 seconds, shake your arms out and then repeat.

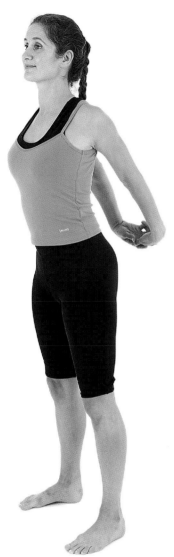

◀ **Chest stretch**

Instructions

1 Stand tall and link your hands together behind your back.

2 Tighten the abdominals to stop your back arching too much and contract the upper back muscles to lift your arms, slightly, behind you. You will feel the pectoral muscles, which form the front of the chest, being stretched out.

3 Hold this stretch and breathe deeply for 15 seconds. Release and shake out your arms by your sides. Repeat once more.

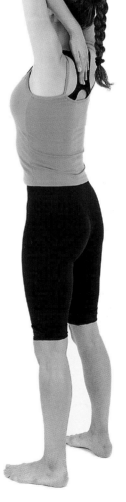

▶ **Tricep press back**

Instructions

1 Stand with good posture and life one arm to drop the hand behind your shoulder.

2 Use the other arm to press the elbow further back, so that you feel a stretch all along the underside of the arm. This is where the tricep muscle is. Don't let your back over-arch as you press your elbow back

3 Hold the stretch for 8–10 seconds. Shake your arms out and repeat on the other arm.

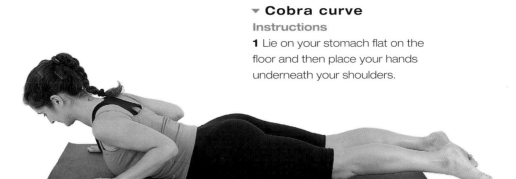

▼ Cobra curve

Instructions

1 Lie on your stomach flat on the floor and then place your hands underneath your shoulders.

2 Now push back on your arms and lift your head and chest upwards and hold. Focus on what you are trying to stretch here – the abdominals. Push back a little further in order to feel the stretch along the front of your body.
3 If your back feels sore during this move, then decrease the stretch slightly.
4 Hold for 8–10 seconds, then rest and repeat

Many people forget that after working their abdominal muscles extremely hard, they need stretching, too.

▼ **Buttock blast**

Instructions

1 Lie on your back and extend your left leg. Now cross your right ankle over the thigh of the straight leg. You will feel a gentle stretch on the outside thigh and buttock of your left leg.

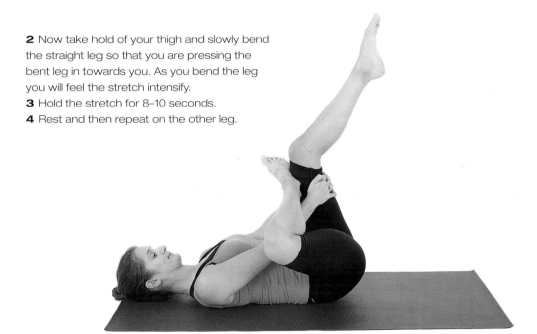

2 Now take hold of your thigh and slowly bend the straight leg so that you are pressing the bent leg in towards you. As you bend the leg you will feel the stretch intensify.

3 Hold the stretch for 8–10 seconds.

4 Rest and then repeat on the other leg.

▼ Quad triangle

When you do this, you'll feel the stretch on the quadriceps muscles on the front of your thighs. If you feel the stretch is enough just by leaning back on your hands, stay in that position.

Instructions

1 Sit on the floor and bend one knee under you with the top of the foot flat on the floor next to your hip. Your other leg is straight out in front.

2 Take your weight behind on your hands and lean back until you can really feel the stretch in the thigh.Hold for 15–20 seconds, then release.

3 Change legs and repeat on the other side. This will stretch the front of the thigh and also the front of the calf.

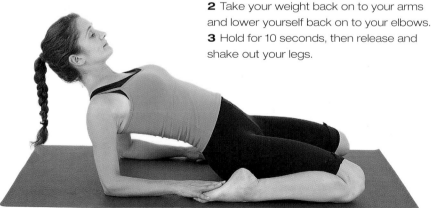

▼ Double leg lean back

Instructions

1 Sit with both legs bent beneath you, the tops of your feet flat on the floor.

2 Take your weight back on to your arms and lower yourself back on to your elbows.

3 Hold for 10 seconds, then release and shake out your legs.

▼ Hamstring triangle

Instructions

1 Sit on the floor with one leg bent out to the side and the other leg straight.

2 Keep your back straight by pulling in on the abdominals and up from your waist.

3 Reach with your hands and lean your body towards the straight leg as far as you can. You will feel the hamstring at the back of the thigh lengthening. The further you lean forwards the greater the stretch.

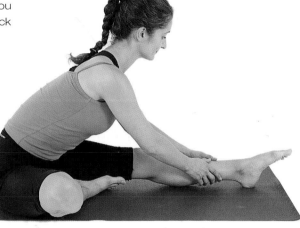

115

4 Put your hands on your leg to ease you forwards and prevent any risk of slipping. You can extend the stretch further by grasping the top of your toes.

5 Hold for 15–20 seconds and then release.

6 Repeat on the other leg.

▼ Hip harp

You will feel this stretch in your hips and legs as you mobilize the hip joints.

Instructions

1 Sit on the floor with one leg bent in front of the other.

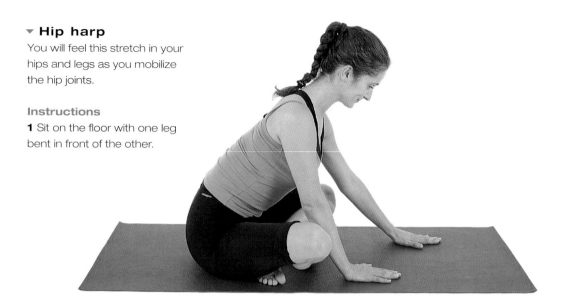

2 Now walk your hands out slowly in front of you so that your body folds over your legs.
3 Hold for 15–20 seconds and then use your hands to walk your body back to upright.

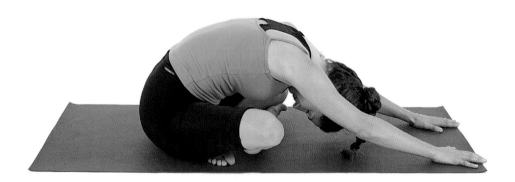

▼ Back walk

Instructions

1 Stand near a wall or a chair. Place your hands on the back of the chair and walk backwards until your back is flat and your legs are at right angles to your torso.

2 Hold this position and allow your head to hang through your arms and your lower back to sink slightly, keeping your abdominals pulled in tightly. You will feel this stretching out the back and shoulders and other places, too!

3 Hold for 15–20 seconds, then walk the feet back in to return to the upright position.

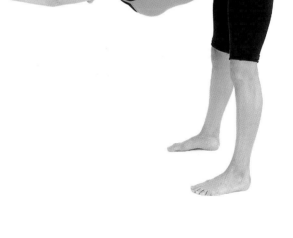

▼ Second stretch

Instructions

1 Sit with your legs apart and extended out to each side. Straigten your back and sit as tall as you possibly can.

2 Now reach forwards with both hands and place them on the ground in front of you. Try to walk your hands forwards as far as possible. You are aiming to take your chest towards the floor as far as you can. Only go as far as feels vaguely uncomfortable and then walk your hands back in again.

3 At the furthest point of your stretch, hold the position for 15 seconds.

4 On releasing the stretch, bend your legs and roll your knees from side to side to relax the muscles.

Your lower legs get used in everyday life and exercise – so stretch them fully.

▶ Calf stretch

You can gently stretch the calf muscles (the gastrocnemius and soleus) to encourage flexibility.

Instructions

1 Stand facing a wall or chair and walk your feet away slightly.

2 Lean forwards until you can place your hands on it. Keep your feet, particularly the heels, on the ground. You will feel the stretch on the back of your calves as you lean forwards.

3 Hold for 15–20 seconds for a really thorough stretch.

4 In this same position, if you bend both knees very slightly, you will focus the stretch on the Achilles tendons. Hold and then shake out.

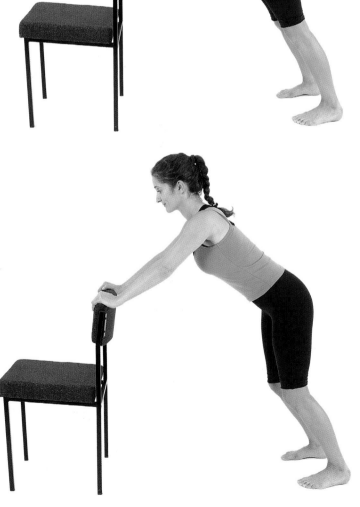

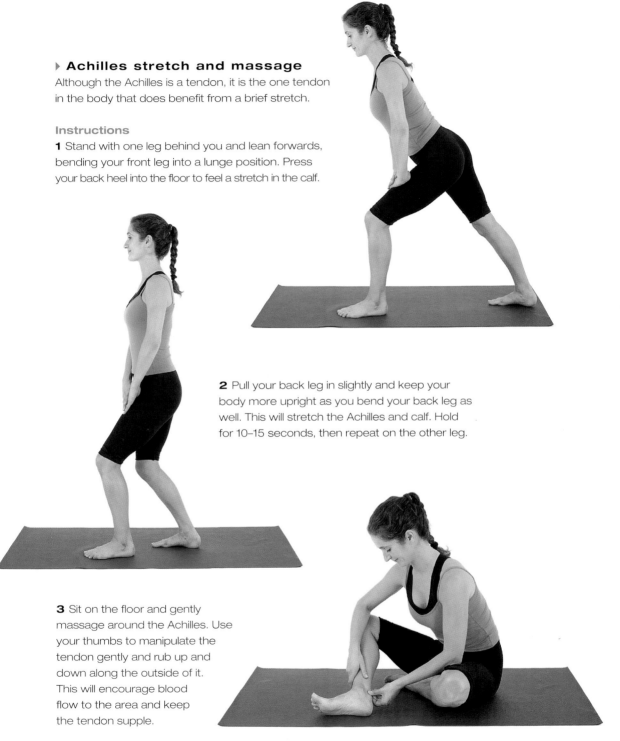

▶ Achilles stretch and massage

Although the Achilles is a tendon, it is the one tendon in the body that does benefit from a brief stretch.

Instructions

1 Stand with one leg behind you and lean forwards, bending your front leg into a lunge position. Press your back heel into the floor to feel a stretch in the calf.

2 Pull your back leg in slightly and keep your body more upright as you bend your back leg as well. This will stretch the Achilles and calf. Hold for 10–15 seconds, then repeat on the other leg.

3 Sit on the floor and gently massage around the Achilles. Use your thumbs to manipulate the tendon gently and rub up and down along the outside of it. This will encourage blood flow to the area and keep the tendon supple.

office workout

In the office it is easy to get involved in what you're doing and forget to get up and move around. If you can, try to build some small activity in to your routine every hour. Not only will this help your body, preventing you from getting too stiff, but it will help relax your mind, too. You will get a break from thinking about any problems you might be dealing with as you focus, briefly, on the exercise, and it will also bring blood to the brain, boosting your mental powers!

▶ Roll down

This will mobilize your back, stretch your lower back and hamstrings and send blood to your brain!

Instructions

1 Push your chair away from your desk and enliven your spine! Gently fold your neck into your chest and let your upper body follow as you curl down.

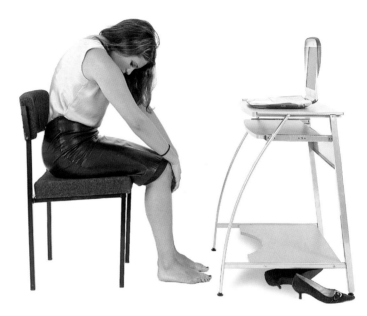

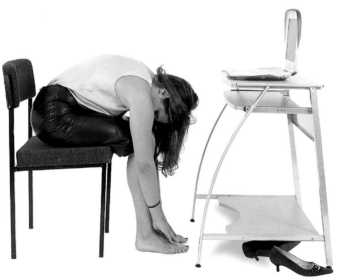

2 Curl all the way over until you can rest your body over your legs. Let your head hang and breathe deeply for 5 breaths.
3 Uncurl your body slowly to return to the starting upright position.
4 Do this every hour.

▼ Chair squats

Do this simple exercise every few
hours at work and, before you know
it, you will have tightened up your
buttocks and thighs beautifully!

Instructions
1 Stand up from your desk
and push your chair away
from you just slightly.

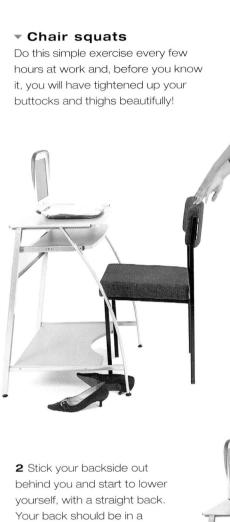

2 Stick your backside out
behind you and start to lower
yourself, with a straight back.
Your back should be in a
straight line from the hips to
the shoulders.
3 Hold, breathing deeply, for
a count of 5. Squeeze your
buttocks to keep the position.
4 Perform 12 lowers and lifts
to really feel the muscles
working!

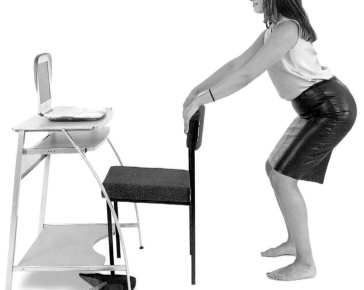

▼ Leg extensions

This simple exercise will tone the front of your legs – the quadriceps muscles.

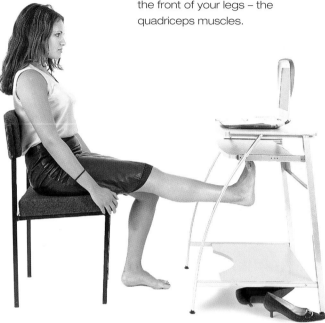

Instructions

1 Push your chair away from your desk and sit upright.

2 Now simply press your knees together and then straighten one leg until your toe touches the underneath of your desk.

3 Press the desk with your toe and then bend your leg back down, contracting the front of the thigh.

4 Repeat 15–20 times to feel the quadriceps really working and then do the same on the other leg.

▶ Seat Salsa

Instructions

1 Sit forward on your chair and, keeping your feet fixed in place, slowly twist around with your upper body until you can place both hands on the back of the chair.

2 Feel the twist in your torso as you breathe and then return to the front.

3 Now repeat the exercise, twisting the other way. Repeat twice on both sides.

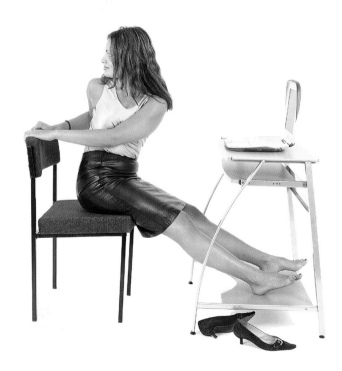

▶ Desk push ups

Instructions

1 Push your chair aside and place your hands on the edge of your desk while you walk your legs backwards.

2 For this exercise you need to keep your legs and your back straight by holding your stomach tense. Now bend your arms, taking your weight with you, as you push up and down. Try to do 20 of these.

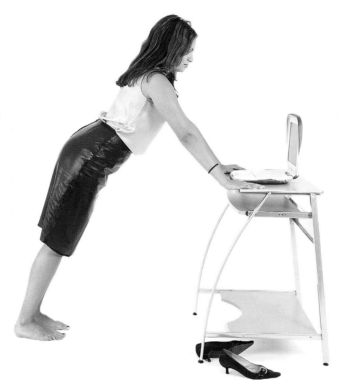

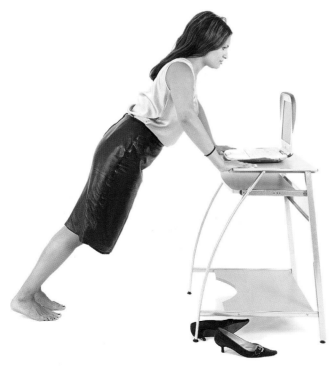

3 This will tone your arms and chest – and wake you up!

cool down

Now that you have completed your 10-minute workout, it's time to do your cool down phase. Think of this as your reward. You have just worked hard, even if only for 10 minutes. Don't forget that this 10 minutes every day of every week of every year will make such a difference to your body and how you feel about it as the years go by.

▶ Knee roll

Instructions

1 Lie on the floor with your knees bent and arms outstretched to the side. Take a few moments just to relax and breathe.

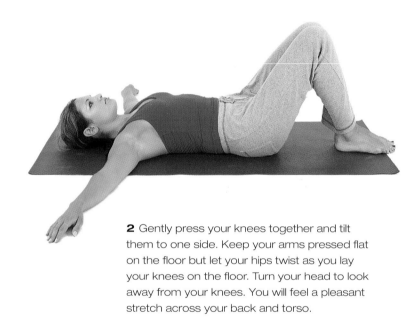

2 Gently press your knees together and tilt them to one side. Keep your arms pressed flat on the floor but let your hips twist as you lay your knees on the floor. Turn your head to look away from your knees. You will feel a pleasant stretch across your back and torso.

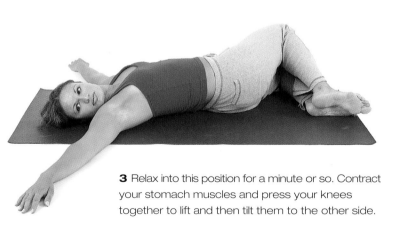

3 Relax into this position for a minute or so. Contract your stomach muscles and press your knees together to lift and then tilt them to the other side.

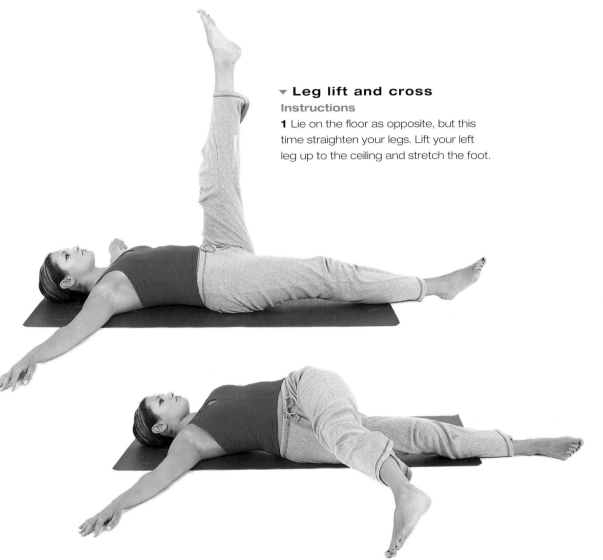

▼ Leg lift and cross

Instructions

1 Lie on the floor as opposite, but this time straighten your legs. Lift your left leg up to the ceiling and stretch the foot.

2 Now slowly lower your leg across your body and take it down towards your right hand. Use your abdominal muscles to control the movement of the leg until it is all the way down to the floor.

3 If you find you are not flexible enough to take your foot all the way to the floor, then bend your left arm up to meet the foot and rest it on your hand.

4 Hold this position for a minute and then carefully lift the leg back to the centre and lower it. Repeat with the other leg.

▼ Double knee hug

Instructions

1 Lie on your back with your legs straight on the floor. Contract your abdominals and pull both legs into your chest. Stay like this, breathing deeply for a few moments.

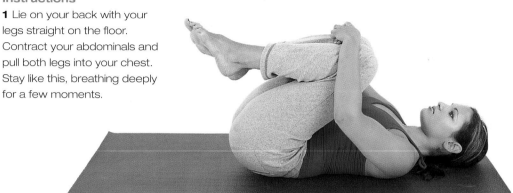

2 Now taking hold of your knees, breathe in and, as you breathe out, hug your knees in tighter to your chest.

3 Release the pull and breathe in, then breathe out and pull in your knees tightly again. Repeat as many times, as you like.

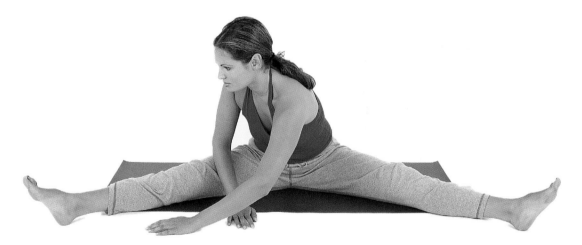

▼ Straddle stretch

Instructions

1 Sit upright with your legs as far apart as possible. Lean forwards with your hands on the floor.
2 Start to walk your hands forwards as far as you can, lowering your chest towards the floor. You will feel the stretch between your legs, but this should feel pleasant and not too painful!

3 Hold the stretch for 15–20 seconds and then slowly walk your hands back in to your body again.
4 Now walk your hands towards one foot, then the other and then back to the centre
5 Each time you do this exercise you'll find that you will stretch a little further.

▼ Leg circles

Instructions

1 Lie on the floor with one knee bent and the foot on the floor and the other leg extended to the ceiling.

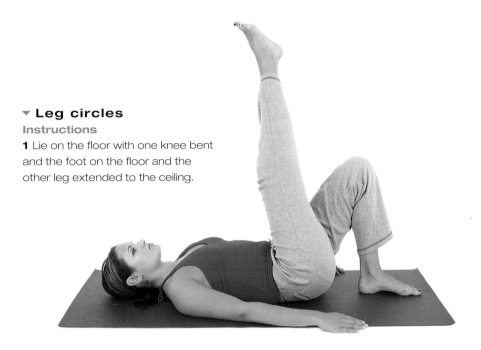

2 Slowly circle your left leg in the hip socket. Gently move the leg as if you are drawing a circle with your toe on the ceiling 8 times, first one way and then the other.

3 This is a gentle mobility exercise for the hips, which will relax you.

4 Repeat this with the other leg.

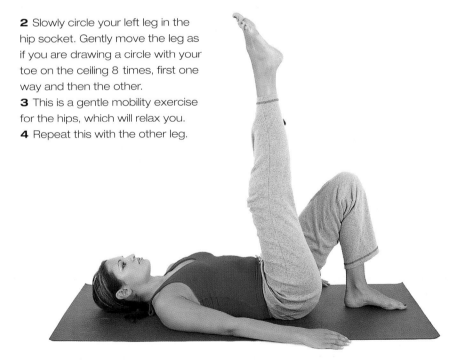

index